Cellular Physiology
of Nerve and Muscle

THIRD EDITION

Cellular Physiology of Nerve and Muscle

Gary G. Matthews

Department of Neurobiology
State University of New York
at Stony Brook

**Blackwell
Science**

©1998 by Blackwell Science, Inc.

Editorial Offices:

350 Main Street, Malden,
  MA 02148-5018, USA

Osney Mead, Oxford OX2 0EL, England

25 John Street, London WC1N 2BL,
  England

23 Ainslie Place, Edinburgh EH3 6AJ,
  Scotland

54 University Street, Carlton,
  Victoria 3053, Australia

Other Editorial Offices:

Blackwell Wissenschafts-Verlag GmbH
  Kurfürstendamm 57
  10707 Berlin, Germany

Blackwell Science KK
  MG Kodenmacho Building
  7–10 Kodenmacho Nihombashi
  Chuo-ku, Tokyo 104, Japan

Distributors

Marston Book Services Ltd
PO Box 269
Abingdon, Oxon OX14 4YN, England
(*Orders:* Tel: 44-01235-465500
  Fax: 44-01235-465555)

USA

Blackwell Science, Inc.
Commerce Place
350 Main Street
Malden, MA 02148-5018
(*Orders:* Tel: 800-759-6102
              617-388-8250
  Fax: 617-388-8255)

Canada

Copp Clark Professional
200 Adelaide Street, West, 3rd Floor
Toronto, Ontario M5H 1W7
(*Orders:* Tel: 800-815-9417
              416-597-1616
  Fax: 416-597-1617)

Australia

Blackwell Science Pty Ltd
54 University Street
Carlton, Victoria 3053
(*Orders:* Tel: 3-9347-0300
  Fax: 3-9349 3016)

Acquisitions: Jane Humphreys
Production: Kevin Sullivan
Manufacturing: Lisa Flanagan
Typeset by Northeastern Graphic Services, Inc.
Printed and bound by Edwards Brothers

Printed in the United States of America
97 98 99 00 5 4 3 2 1

The Blackwell Science logo is a trade mark of Blackwell Science Ltd, registered at the United Kingdom Trade Marks Registry

Library of Congress Cataloging-in-Publication Data

Matthews, Gary G., 1949–
    Cellular physiology of nerve and muscle / Gary G. Matthews.—
    3rd ed.
        p. cm.
    Includes bibliographical references and index.
    ISBN 0-632-04354-7
    1. Neurons. 2. Muscle cells. 3. Nerves—Cytology. 4. Muscles—
    Cytology. I. Title.
    [DNLM: 1. Membrane Potentials—physiology. 2. Neurons—
    cytology. 3. Cell Membrane—physiology. 4. Action Potentials—
    physiology. 5. Muscles—cytology. 6. Synaptic Transmission—
    physiology. WL 102.5 M439c 1997]
    QP363.M38 1997
    573.8'36—dc21
    DNLM/DLC
    for Library of Congress   97-14314
                                                                    CIP

Contents

Part III: Cellular Physiology of Muscle Cells   171

Preface

This book focuses on the electrical behavior of nerve and muscle cells. It is intended to introduce the subject to students who have completed an introductory biology course and who understand a few basic facts about chemistry and physics. It is not intended, however, to be a comprehensive survey of nerve and muscle physiology. Rather, I have limited the material for the most part to the basic physical and chemical principles underlying the functioning of neurons and muscle cells. In my experience as a teacher, the electrical mechanisms of excitable cells are among the most difficult topics for biology students to master. Part of the problem is that beginning students have difficulty extracting the basic principles from the array of facts and experimental results inherent in a comprehensive presentation of nerve–muscle physiology. My approach circumvents this problem by using a series of simplified models and schematic distillations of experimental results, each tailored to illustrate a particular principle. I have included descriptions of actual experiments when I think they might be interesting or provide an especially good example, but for the most part I construct hypothetical experiments and models to focus attention on the particular point at hand. Similarly, I have not shied from quantitative material when it is necessary and can be integrated into a developing presentation of a topic, but I have not included equations for their own sake.

In this edition, I have expanded the coverage of molecular properties of ion channels and the description of neurotransmitter actions mediated via intracellular second messengers. The neural control of the heart is used as an example system in the expanded discussion of second-messenger actions. This addition also serves to introduce the autonomic nervous system, which represents a major new topic in the third edition. I have also expanded and updated the list of suggested readings.

The positive response to the first two editions of this book has been very gratifying. In particular, the approach used here for teaching the basic electrical properties of cells—based on simplified models to illustrate the underlying principles—has proven to be quite successful. I hope that both instructors and students will continue to find this third edition a useful introduction to cellular aspects of neurobiology and muscle physiology. I would also like to point out that I have recently written a general introduction to neurobiology, called *Neurobiology: Molecules, Cells, and Systems*, which is also published by Blackwell Science. The philosophy of that book mirrors that applied here, and I hope it will be similarly useful for students interested in a more comprehensive treatment of neurobiology.

ORIGIN OF ELECTRICAL MEMBRANE POTENTIAL

This book is about some of the physiological characteristics of nerve and muscle cells. As we shall see, many of the important functions of these cells are carried out by electrical mechanisms. That is, the properties of these cells as generators and conductors of electricity are vital to their functioning. Our goal, then, is to arrive at an understanding of the basic physical and chemical principles underlying the electrical behavior of nerve and muscle cells and to apply those principles to the normal physiologic functioning of those cells in the body.

Because an understanding of how electrical voltages and currents arise in cells is central to this book, Part I is devoted to this task. The discussion begins with a presentation of the differences in the composition of the fluids found inside and outside cells. We then consider the factors that are important in achieving osmotic and electrochemical equilibrium states, given the differences between the intracellular and extracellular fluids. We then learn that animal cells are not at equilibrium, but rather must expend energy in order to maintain the differing compositions of their internal and external fluids. By the end of Part I, we will arrive at a quantitative description of the relation between ionic gradients and electrical gradients across cell membranes. This quantitative description sets the stage for the specific descriptions of nerve and muscle cells in the remaining chapters of the book and is central to understanding how the nervous system functions as a transmitter of electrical signals.

Part II of the book examines cellular properties of individual nerve cells and the interactions among nerve cells, again emphasizing the electrical properties developed in Part I. Part III concerns muscle cells and their control by the nervous system. In this case, however, the emphasis is on the linkage between the electrical signal in a single muscle and the mechanical contraction and on the mechanical properties that are important in the regulation of contraction by the nervous system. Part III also describes the electrical differences between the muscle cells of the heart and those of other muscles and relates these differences to the specialized function of the heart muscle.

Throughout the book, little is assumed in terms of background knowledge in physics, chemistry, or mathematics. Important quantitative principles are derived from examples and are explained in a qualitative as well as quantitative manner. It is assumed, however, that the reader has completed an introductory, college-level course in biology and understands the basic characteristics of cells and cellular metabolism.

Composition of Intracellular and Extracellular Fluids

When we think of biological molecules, we normally think of all the special molecules that are unique to living organisms, such as proteins and nucleic acids: enzymes, DNA, RNA, and so on. These are the substances that allow life to occur and that give living things their special characteristics. Yet, if we were to dissociate a human body into its component molecules and sort them by type, we would find that these special molecules are only a small minority of the total. Of all the molecules in a human body, only about 0.25% fall within the category of these special biological molecules. Most of the molecules are far more ordinary. In fact, the most common molecule in the body is water. Excluding non-essential body fat, water makes up about 75% of the weight of a human body. Because water is a comparatively light molecule, especially when compared with massive protein molecules, this 75% of body weight translates into a staggering number of molecules of water. Thus, water accounts for about 99% of all molecules in the body. The remaining 0.75% consists of other simple inorganic substances, mostly sodium, potassium, and chloride ions. In the first part of this book, we are concerned in large part with the mundane majority of molecules, the 99.75% made up of water and inorganic ions.

Why should we study these mundane molecules? Although many enzymatic reactions involving the more glamorous organic molecules require the participation of inorganic cofactors, and although most biochemical reactions within cells occur among substances that are dissolved in water, most inorganic molecules in the body never participate in any biochemical reactions. In spite of this, a sufficient reason to study these substances is that cells could not exist and life as we know it would not be possible if cells did not possess mechanisms to control the distribution of water and ions across their membranes. The purpose of the first four chapters of this book is to see why that is true and to understand the physical principles that underlie the ability of cells to maintain their integrity in a hostile physicochemical environment.

Intracellular and Extracellular Fluids

The water in the body can be divided into two compartments: intracellular and extracellular fluid. About 55% of the water is inside cells, and the remainder is outside. The extracellular fluid, or ECF, can in turn be subdivided into plasma, lymphatic fluid, and interstitial fluid, but for now we can lump all the ECF together into one compartment. Similarly, there are subcompartments within cells, but it will suffice for now to treat cells as uniform bags of fluid. The wall that separates the intracellular and extracellular fluid compartments is the outer cell membrane, also called the **plasma membrane** of the cell.

There are both organic and inorganic substances dissolved in the intracellular and extracellular water, but the compositions of the two fluid compartments are different. Table 1-1 gives simplified compositions of ECF and intracellular fluid (ICF) for a typical mammalian cell. The table is simplified because it includes only those substances that are important in governing the basic osmotic and electrical properties of cells. There are many more kinds of inorganic and organic solutes in both ECF and ICF, and many of them have important physiological roles in other contexts. For the present, however, they can be safely ignored.

The principal cation (positively charged ion) outside the cell is sodium, although there is a small amount of potassium, which will be important to consider when we discuss the origin of the membrane potential of cells. Inside cells, the situation is very different. In ICF, the principal cation is potassium, although there is a small amount of sodium. Negatively charged chloride ions, which are present at high concentration in ECF, are relatively scarce in ICF. The major anion (negatively charged ion) inside cells is actually a class of molecules that bear a net negative charge. These intracellular anions, which we abbreviate as A^-, include protein molecules, acidic amino acids like aspartate and glutamate, and inorganic ions like sulfate and phosphate. For the purposes of this

Table 1-1   Simplified compositions of intracellular and extracellular fluids for a typical mammalian cell.

	Internal concentration (m*M*)	External concentration (m*M*)	Can it cross plasma membrane?
K^+	125	5	Y
Na^+	12	120	N*
Cl^-	5	125	Y
A^-	108	0	N
H_2O	55,000	55,000	Y
	Membrane potential = −60 to −100 mV		

*As we will see in Chapter 3, this No is not as simple as it first appears.

book, the anions of this class outside cells can be ignored; we will say that the only extracellular anion is chloride.

It is also important to consider the concentration of water on the two sides of the membrane, which is also shown in Table 1-1. It may seem odd to speak of the "concentration" of the solvent in ECF and ICF. However, as we will see when we consider the maintenance of cell volume, the concentration of water inside and outside the cell must be the same or water will move across the membrane and cell volume will change.

Another important consideration is whether or not a particular substance can cross the plasma membrane—that is, whether the membrane is permeable to that substance. The plasma membrane is permeable to water, potassium, and chloride, but is effectively impermeable to sodium (however, more will be said about sodium permeability later). Of course, if the membrane is to do its job properly, it must keep the organic anions inside the cell; otherwise all of a cell's essential biochemical machinery would simply diffuse away into the ECF. Thus, the membrane is impermeable to A^-.

An ultrafine probe, called an intracellular microelectrode, can be inserted inside an animal cell to measure the electrical voltage difference between the inside and outside of the cell. The inside is more negative than the outside. The difference is usually about 60 to 100 millivolts (mV), and is referred to as the **membrane potential** of the cell. By convention, the potential outside the cell is called zero; therefore, the typical value of the membrane potential (abbreviated E_m) is −60 to −100 mV, as shown in Table 1-1. A major concern of the first section of this book is the origin of this electrical membrane potential. In later sections, we discuss how the membrane potential influences the movement of charged particles across the cell membrane and how the electrical energy stored in the membrane potential can be tapped to generate signals that can be passed from one cell to another in the nervous system.

The Structure of the Plasma Membrane

Before we consider the mechanisms that allow cells to maintain the differences in ECF and ICF shown in Table 1-1, it is helpful to look at the structure of the outer membrane of the cell, the plasma membrane. The control mechanisms responsible for the differences between ICF and ECF reside within that barrier between the intracellular and extracellular compartments.

It has long been known that the contents of a cell will leak out if the cell is damaged by being poked or prodded with a glass probe. Also, when dissolved in the ECF some dyes will not enter cells, and when injected inside cells the same dyes will not leak out. These observations, first made in the nineteenth century, led to the idea that there is a selectively permeable barrier—the plasma membrane—separating the intracellular and extracellular fluid.

The first systematic observations of the kinds of molecules that would enter cells and the kinds that were excluded were made by Overton in the early part of the twentieth century. He found that, in general, substances that are highly soluble in lipids enter cells more easily than do substances that are less soluble in lipids. Lipids are molecules that are not soluble in water or other polar solvents, but are soluble in oil or other nonpolar solvents. Thus, Overton suggested that the plasma membrane of a cell is made of lipids and that substances can cross the membrane if they can dissolve in that lipid barrier.

There were some exceptions to the general lipid solubility rule. Electrically charged substances, like potassium and chloride ions, are almost totally insoluble in lipids, yet they manage to cross the plasma membrane. Other substances, such as urea, entered cells more easily than might be expected based on their lipid solubility alone. To take account of these exceptions, Overton suggested that the lipid membrane is shot through with tiny holes or pores that allow highly water-soluble (hydrophilic) substances, such as ions, to cross the membrane. Only hydrophilic substances that are small enough to fit through these small aqueous pores can cross the membrane. Larger molecules like proteins and amino acids cannot fit through the pores and thus cannot cross the membrane without the help of special transport mechanisms.

The molecules of the lipid skin of cell membranes appear to be arranged in a layer only two molecules thick. Evidence for this arrangement was obtained from experiments in which the lipids were chemically extracted from the plasma membranes of cells and spread out on a trough of water in such a way that they formed a film only one molecule thick. When the area of this monolayer "oil slick" was measured, it was found to be about twice the total surface area of the intact cells from which the lipids were obtained. This suggests that the membrane of the intact cells was two molecules thick. Such a membrane is called a lipid bilayer membrane.

The bilayer arrangement of the cell membrane makes chemical sense when we consider the characteristics of the kinds of lipid molecules found in the plasma membrane. The cell lipids are largely phospholipids, which are molecules that have both a polar region that is hydrophilic and a nonpolar region that is hydrophobic. When surrounded by water, these lipid molecules tend to aggregate, with the hydrophilic regions oriented out toward the surrounding water and the hydrophobic regions pointed toward each other. When spread out in a sheet with water on each side of the sheet, the phospholipids can maintain their preferred state by forming a bimolecular sandwich, with the hydrophilic parts on the outside pointed toward the water and the hydrophobic parts in the middle pointed toward each other. This bilayer model for the cell plasma membrane is illustrated in Figure 1-1.

Figure 1-1 also shows another important characteristic of cell membranes. They contain not only lipid molecules but also protein molecules. Some proteins are attached to the inner or outer surface of the cell membrane, and others penetrate all the way through the membrane so that they form a bridge from one side to the other. Some of the transmembrane proteins form the aqueous pores, or channels, that allow ions and other small hydrophilic molecules to cross the membrane. If we separate membranes from the rest of the cell and analyze their composition, we find that, by weight, only about one-third of the membrane material is lipid; most of the rest is protein. Thus, the lipids form the backbone of the membrane, but proteins are an important part of the picture. We will see later that the proteins are very important

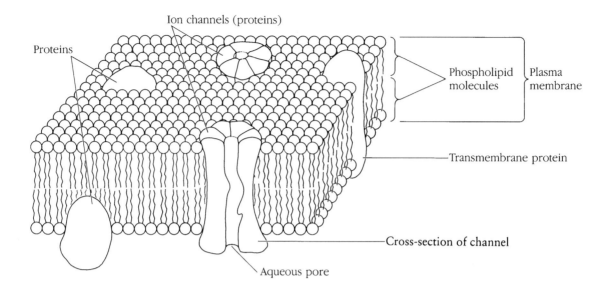

Figure 1-1
Schematic diagram of a section of the plasma membrane. The backbone of the membrane is a sheet of lipid molecules two molecules thick. Inserted into this sheet are various types of protein molecules. Some protein molecules extend all the way across the sheet from the inner to the outer face. These transmembrane proteins sometimes form small-diameter aqueous pores or channels through which small hydrophilic molecules, such as ions, can cross the membrane. In the diagram, two such channels are shown, one cut in cross-section to reveal the interior of the pore.

in controlling the movement of substances, particularly ions, across the cell membrane.

We can get an idea of the importance of membrane proteins for life by examining how much of the entire genome of a simple organism is taken up by genes encoding membrane proteins. One of the smallest genomes of any free-living organism is that of *Mycoplasma genitalium*, a microbe whose genome can be regarded as close to the minimum required for an independent, cellular life form. The DNA of *M. genitalium* has been completely sequenced, revealing a total of 482 individual genes. Of this total, 140 genes, or about 30%, code for membrane proteins. Thus, *M. genitalium* expends a large fraction of its total available DNA for the membrane proteins that sit at the interface between the microbe and its external environment. This points out the central role of these proteins in the maintenance of cellular life.

Anatomical evidence also supports the model shown in Figure 1-1. The cell membrane is much too thin to be seen with the light microscope. In fact, it is almost too thin to be seen with the electron microscope. However, with an electron microscope it is possible to see at the outer boundary of a cell a three-layered (trilaminar) profile similar to a railroad track, with a light region separating two darker bands. Figure 1-2 is an example of an electron micrograph showing the plasma membranes of two cells lying in close contact. The interpretation of the trilaminar profile is that the two dark

0.1 μm

Figure 1-2

High-power electron micrograph of the plasma membranes of two neighboring cells. Note the two dark bands separated by a light region at the outer surface of each cell. The two cells are nerve cells from the brain, and the point of close contact between them is a **synapse**, the point of information transfer in the nervous system. Note also the membrane-bound intracellular structures (labeled SV), called **synaptic vesicles**, inside one of the cells; the vesicle membranes also have the trilaminar profile seen in the plasma membranes. We will learn more about synaptic vesicles and synapses in Chapters 7 and 8. (Courtesy of A. L. deBlas of the University of Missouri, Kansas City.)

bands represent the polar heads of the membrane phospholipids and protein molecules on the inner and outer surfaces of the membrane and that the lighter region between the two dark bands represents the nonpolar tails of the lipid molecules. The total thickness of the sandwich is about 7.5 nm. The lighter-colored "fuzz" surrounding the trilaminar profiles of the two cell membranes in Figure 1-2 consists in part of portions of membrane-associated protein molecules extending out into the intracellular and extracellular spaces. The two cells shown in Figure 1-2 are nerve cells (neurons) in the brain, and the region of close contact is a specialized junction, called a synapse, where electrical activity is relayed from one nerve cell to another. One of our major goals in this book is to understand how such synapses, the basic mechanism of information transfer in the brain, work.

By using a special form of microscopy called freeze-fracture electron microscopy, it is possible to visualize more clearly the protein molecules that are embedded in the plasma membrane. A schematic representation of the freeze-fracture technique is shown

Figure 1-3
Schematic illustration of the freeze-fracture procedure for electron microscopy. When a fracture line runs between the two lipid layers of the plasma membrane, some membrane proteins stay with one monolayer, and others with the other layer. If the fractured surface is then examined with the electron microscope, the remaining proteins appear as protruding bumps in the surface.

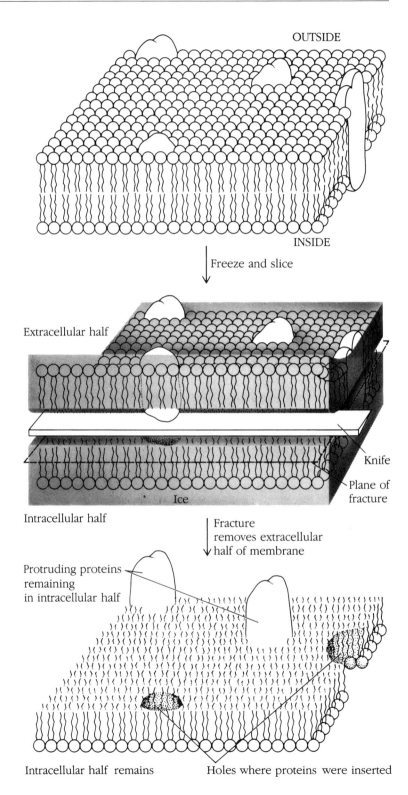

OUTSIDE

INSIDE

Freeze and slice

Extracellular half

Knife

Plane of fracture

Intracellular half

Ice

Fracture removes extracellular half of membrane

Protruding proteins remaining in intracellular half

Intracellular half remains

Holes where proteins were inserted

0.5 μm

Figure 1-4
Example of a fractured membrane surface containing protein molecules, viewed through the electron microscope. The membrane surface shown is that of the presynaptic nerve terminal at the nerve-muscle junction, which is discussed in detail in Chapter 7. The protein molecules are the small bumps scattered about on the planar surface of the membrane. (Reproduced from Ko C.-P. Regeneration of the active zone at the frog neuromuscular junction. *Cell Biol* 1984;98: 1685–1695 by copyright permission of the Rockefeller University Press.)

in Figure 1-3. A small sample of the tissue to be examined is frozen in liquid nitrogen, and then a thin sliver of the frozen tissue is shaved off with a sharp knife. Because the tissue is frozen, however, the sliver is not so much sliced off as broken off from the sample. In some cases, like that shown in Figure 1-3, the line of fracture runs between the two lipid layers of the membrane bilayer, leaving holes where protein molecules are ripped out of the lipid monolayer and protrusions where membrane proteins are ripped out of the opposing monolayer and come along with the shaved sliver. An example of such a freeze-fracture sample viewed through the electron microscope is shown in Figure 1-4. The membrane proteins appear as small bumps in the otherwise smooth surface of the plasma membrane, like grains of sand sprinkled on a freshly painted surface. In the discussion of the transmission of signals from one nerve cell to another in Chapter 7, we show other examples of freeze-fracture electron micrographs and see how they can provide important evidence about the physiological functioning of cells.

Summary

The most common molecules in the body are water and simple inorganic molecules—mainly sodium, potassium, and chloride ions. The water in the body can be divided into two compartments: the intracellular and extracellular fluids. The barrier between these two compartments is the plasma membrane of the cell, which is a phospholipid bilayer with protein molecules inserted into it. The ECF is high in sodium and chloride, but low in potassium, while the ICF is low in sodium and chloride, but high in potassium. This difference is maintained and regulated by control mechanisms residing in the plasma membrane, which acts as a selectively permeable barrier permitting some substances to cross but excluding others.

2

Maintenance of Cell Volume

At an early stage of evolution, before the development of cells, life might well have been nothing more than a loose confederation of enzyme systems and self-replicating molecules. A major problem faced by such acellular systems must have been how to keep their constituent parts from simply diffusing away into the surrounding murk. The solution to this problem was the development of a cell membrane that was impermeable to these organic molecules; this was the origin of cellular life. However, the cell membrane, while solving one problem, brought with it a new problem: how to achieve osmotic balance. To see how this problem arises, we begin with a review of solutions, osmolarity, and osmosis. We then analyze the cellular mechanisms used to deal with problems of osmotic balance.

Molarity, Molality, and Diffusion of Water

Examine the situation illustrated in Figure 2-1. We take 1 liter of pure water and dissolve some sugar in it. The dissolved sugar molecules take up some space that was formerly occupied by water molecules, and thus the volume of the solution increases. Recall that the concentration of a substance is defined as the number of molecules of that substance per unit volume of solution. As shown in Figure 2-1, this means that the concentration of water in the sugar-water solution is lower than it was before the sugar was dissolved. This is because the total volume increased after the sugar was added, but the total number of water molecules

Figure 2-1
When sugar molecules (filled circles) are dissolved in 1 liter of water, the resulting solution occupies a volume greater than 1 liter. This is because the sugar molecules have taken up some space formerly occupied by water molecules (open circles). Therefore, the concentration of water (number of molecules of water per unit volume) is lower in the sugar-water solution.

present was the same before and after the sugar dissolved in the water.

In order to compare the concentrations of water in solutions containing different concentrations of dissolved substances, we will use the concept of **osmolarity**. A solution containing 1 mole of dissolved particles per liter of solution (a 1 molar, or 1 M, solution) is said to have an osmolarity of 1 osmolar (1 Osm), and a 1 millimolar (1 mM) solution has an osmolarity of 1 milliosmolar (1 mOsm). *The higher the osmolarity of a solution, the lower the concentration of water.* For practical purposes in biological solutions, it doesn't matter what the dissolved particle is; that is, the concentration of water is effectively the same in a solution of 0.1 Osm glucose, 0.1 Osm sucrose, or 0.1 Osm urea. To be strictly correct in discussing the concentration of water in various solutions, we would have to speak of the **molality**, rather than the molarity, of the solutions. Whereas molarity is defined as moles of solute per liter of solution, molality is defined as moles of solute per kilogram of solvent. This means that molality takes into account the fact that higher-molecular-weight solutes displace more water per mole of solute than do lower-molecular-weight solutes. That is, 1 liter of solution containing 1 mole of a large molecule, like a protein, would contain less water than 1 liter of solution containing 1 mole of a small molecule, like urea. Thus, the molality of the protein solution would be higher than the molality of the urea solution, even though both solutions have the same molarity (1 M). For our purposes in this book, however, it is adequate to treat molarity and osmolarity as equivalent to molality and osmolality.

It is important in determining the osmolarity of a solution to take into account how many dissolved particles result from each molecule of the dissolved substance. Glucose, sucrose, and urea molecules don't dissociate when they dissolve, and thus a 0.1 M glucose solution is a 0.1 Osm solution. A solution of sodium chloride (NaCl), however, contains two dissolved particles—a sodium and a chloride ion—from each molecule of salt that goes into solution. Thus, a 0.1 M NaCl solution is a 0.2 Osm solution. To be strictly correct, we would have to take into account interactions among the ions in a solution, so that the effective osmolarity might be less than we would expect from assuming that all dissolved particles behave independently. But for dilute solutions like those we usually encounter in cell biology, such interactions are weak and can be safely ignored. Thus, for practical purposes we assume that all dissolved particles act independently in determining the total osmolarity of a solution. This means that solutions containing 300 mM glucose, 150 mM NaCl, 100 mM NaCl + 100 mM glucose, or 75 mM NaCl + 75 mM KCl would all have the same total osmolarity—300 mOsm.

When solutions of different osmolarity are placed in contact through a barrier that allows water to move across, water will diffuse across the barrier down its concentration gradient (that is, from the lower osmolar solution to the higher). This movement of water down its concentration gradient is called osmosis. Consider the example shown in Figure 2-2A, which shows a container divided into two equal compartments that are filled with glucose solutions. Imagine that the barrier dividing the container is made of an elastic material, so that it can stretch freely. If the barrier allows both water and glucose to cross, then water will move from side 1 to side 2, down its concentration gradient, and glucose will move from side 2 to side 1. The movement of water and glucose will continue until their concentrations on the two sides of the barrier are equal. Thus, side 1 gains glucose and loses water, and side 2 loses glucose and gains water until the glucose concentration on both sides is 150 mM. There will be no net change in the volume of solution on either side of the barrier, as shown in Figure 2-2B.

If the barrier in Figure 2-2A allows water but not glucose to cross, however, the outcome will be quite different from that shown in Figure 2-2B. Once again, water will move down its concentration gradient from side 1 to side 2. In this case, though, the loss of water will not be compensated by a gain of glucose. As water continues to leave side 1 and accumulates on side 2, the volume of side 2 will increase and the volume of side 1 will decrease. The accumulating water will exert a pressure on the elastic barrier, causing it to expand to the left to accommodate the volume changes (as shown in Figure 2-2C). The resulting volume changes will increase the osmolarity of side 1 and decrease the osmolarity of side 2, and this will continue until the osmolarities

Figure 2-2
Effect of the properties of the barrier separating two different glucose solutions (A) on the final volumes of the solutions. (B) If the barrier allows both glucose and water to cross, the volumes of the two solutions do not change when equilibrium is reached. (C) If the barrier allows only water to cross, osmolarities of the two solutions are again the same at equilibrium, but the final volumes are different.

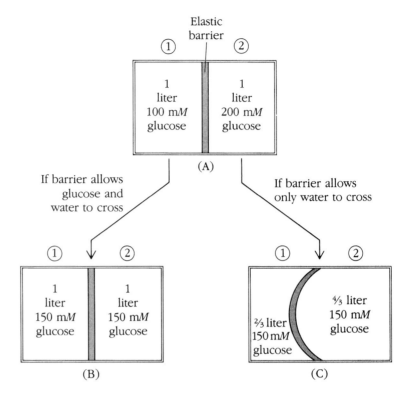

of the two sides are equal—150 mOsm. To prevent the changes in volume, we would have to exert a pressure against the elastic barrier from side 1 to keep it from stretching. This pressure would be equal to the pressure moving water down its concentration gradient and would provide a measure of the **osmotic pressure** gradient across the barrier.

Osmotic Balance and Cell Volume

Return now to the hypothetical primitive cell, early after the development of a cell membrane. In order for the cell membrane to do its job, it must be impermeable to the organic molecules inside the cell. But if the compositions of the extracellular and intracellular fluids are the same, with the exception of the internal organic molecules, the cell faces an imbalance of water on the two sides of the membrane. This is shown schematically in Figure 2-3. Here, the solutes that are in common in ICF and ECF are grouped together and symbolized by S. The extra solute inside the cell—the organic molecules (symbolized by P, for protein)—cause the concentration of water inside the cell to be less than it is outside. Put another way, the total osmolarity inside the cell is greater than it is outside the cell. There are two solutes inside, S and P, and only one outside. Therefore, water will enter the cell and will continue to enter until the osmolarity on the two sides of the membrane is the same. Because the volume of the sea is essentially infinite relative to the volume of a cell and can thus be treated as constant, this end point could be reached only when the internal concentration of organic solutes is zero. This would require the volume of the cell to be infinite. Real cell membranes are not infinitely elastic, and thus water will enter the cell, causing it to swell, until the membrane ruptures and the cell bursts.

   It is convenient to summarize this situation in equation form. *If a substance is at diffusion equilibrium across a cell membrane, there is no net movement of that substance across the membrane.* For any solute, S, that can cross the cell membrane, diffusion equilibrium will be reached when

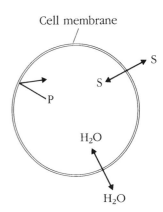

Figure 2-3
A simple model cell containing organic molecules, P. The ECF is a solution of solute, S, in water. Both water and S can cross the cell membrane, but P cannot.

$$[S]_i = [S]_o \qquad (2\text{-}1)$$

The square brackets indicate the concentration of a substance, and the subscripts i and o refer to the inside and outside of the cell. Thus, in order for water to be at equilibrium, we would expect that

$$[S]_i + [P]_i = [S]_o \qquad (2\text{-}2)$$

which is the same as saying that at equilibrium, the total osmolarity inside the cell must be the same as the total osmolarity outside the cell. For the cell represented in Figure 2-3, diffusion equilibrium will be reached only when the concentrations of all substances that can cross the membrane (in this case, S and water) are the same inside and outside the cell. This would require that Equations (2-1) and (2-2) be true simultaneously, which can occur only if $[P]_i$ is zero.

Answers to the Problem of Osmotic Balance

What solutions exist to this apparently fatal problem? There are three basic strategies that have developed in different types of cells. First, the problem could be eliminated by making the cell membrane impermeable to water. This turns out to be quite difficult to do and is not a commonly found solution to the problem of osmotic balance. However, certain kinds of epithelial cells have achieved very low permeability to water. A second strategy is commonly found and was likely the first solution to the problem. Here, the basic idea is to use brute force: Build an inelastic wall around the cell membrane to physically prevent the cell from swelling. This is the solution used by bacteria and plants. The third strategy is that found in animal cells: Achieve osmotic balance by making the cell membrane impermeable to selected extracellular solutes. This solution to the problem of osmotic balance works by balancing the concentration of nonpermeating molecules inside the cell with the same concentration of nonpermeating solutes outside the cell.

To see how the third strategy works, it is useful to work through some examples using a simplified model animal cell whose membrane is permeable to water. Suppose that the model cell contains only one solute: nonpermeating protein molecules, P, dissolved in water at a concentration of 0.25 *M*. We then perform a series of experiments on this model cell by placing it in various ECFs and deducing what would happen to its volume in each case. Assume that the initial volume of the cell is one-billionth of a liter (1 nanoliter, or 1 nl) and that the volume of the ECF in each case is infinite. This latter assumption means that the concentration of extracellular solutes does not change during the experiments.

The first experiment involves placing the cell in a 0.25 *M* solution of sucrose, which does not cross cell membranes. This is shown in Figure 2-4A. In this situation, only water can cross the cell membrane. For water to be at equilibrium, the internal osmolarity must equal the external osmolarity, or

$$[P]_i = [sucrose]_o \qquad (2\text{-}3)$$

Because the internal and external osmolarities are both 0.25 Osm, this condition is met; there will be no net diffusion of water, and cell volume will not change.

In the second example, shown in Figure 2-4B, imagine that the cell is placed in 0.125 *M* sucrose rather than 0.25 *M* sucrose. Again, only water can cross the membrane, and Equation (2-3) must be satisfied for equilibrium to be reached. In 0.125 *M* sucrose, however, the internal osmolarity is greater than the external osmolarity, and water will enter the cell until the internal osmolarity falls to 0.125 *M*. This will happen when the cell volume is twice normal,

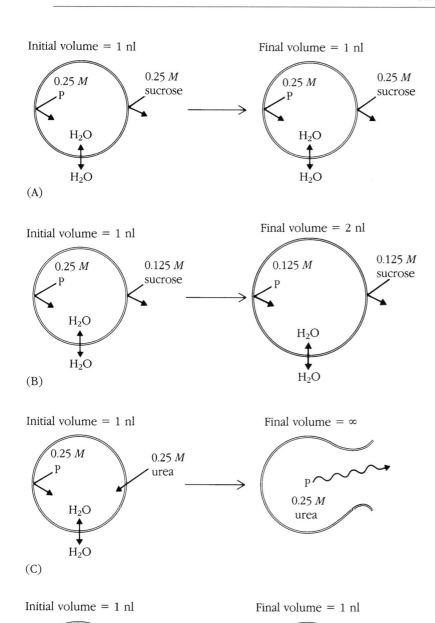

Figure 2-4
Effects of various ECFs on the volume of a simple model. (A) The ECF contains an impermeant solute (sucrose), and the osmolarity is the same as that inside the cell. (B) The ECF contains an impermeant solute, and the osmolarity is lower than that inside the cell. (C) The ECF contains a permeant solute (urea) and external and internal osmolarities are equal. (D) The ECF contains a mixture of permeant and impermeant solutes.

that is, 2 nl. What would the equilibrium cell volume be if we placed the cell in 0.5 M sucrose rather than 0.125 M?

The point of the previous two examples is that *water will be at equilibrium if the concentration of impermeant extracellular solute is the same as the concentration of impermeant internal solute.* To see that the external solute must not be able to cross the cell membrane, consider the example shown in Figure 2-4C. In this case, the model cell is placed in 0.25 M urea, rather than sucrose. Unlike sucrose, urea can cross the cell membrane, and thus we must take into account both urea and water in determining diffusion equilibrium. In equation form, equilibrium will be reached when these two relations hold:

$$[urea]_i = [urea]_o \tag{2-4}$$

$$[urea]_i + [P]_i = [urea]_o \tag{2-5}$$

Because the external volume is infinite, $[urea]_o$ will be 0.25 M at equilibrium, and according to Equation (2-4) $[urea]_i$ will also be 0.25 M. Equations (2-4) and (2-5) require, then, that $[P]_i$ be zero at equilibrium. Thus, the equilibrium volume is infinite, and the cell will swell until it bursts. Qualitatively, when the cell is first placed in 0.25 M urea, there will be no net movement of water across the membrane because internal and external osmolarities are both 0.25 Osm. But as urea enters the cell down its concentration gradient, internal osmolarity rises as urea accumulates. Water will then begin to enter the cell down its concentration gradient. The cell begins to swell and continues to do so until it bursts. Thus, an extracellular solute that can cross the cell membrane cannot help a cell achieve osmotic balance.

An interesting example is shown in Figure 2-4D. In this experiment, the model cell is placed in a mixture of 0.25 M urea and 0.25 M sucrose. The equilibrium for urea will once again be given by Equation (2-4), and water will be at equilibrium when

$$[urea]_i + [P]_i = [urea]_o + [sucrose]_o \tag{2-6}$$

Both Equation (2-4) and Equation (2-6) will be satisfied when $[P]_i$ = 0.25 M, which is the initial condition. Therefore, in this example, the cell volume at diffusion equilibrium will be the normal volume, 1 nl. The point is that even if some extracellular solutes can cross the cell membrane, the presence of a nonpermeating external solute at the same concentration as the nonpermeating internal solute allows the cell to achieve diffusion equilibrium for water and thus to maintain its volume. This is the strategy taken by animal cells to avoid bursting. As shown in Table 1-1, the impermeant extracellular solute is sodium.

In all the examples of osmotic equilibrium we just worked through, the answer was arrived at using just one rule: *For each permeating substance (including water), the inside concentration must equal the outside concentration at equilibrium.*

Tonicity

In the examples in Figure 2-4, 0.25 *M* sucrose and 0.25 *M* urea had the same osmolarity: 0.25 Osm. But the two solutions had dramatically different effects on cell volume. In 0.25 *M* sucrose, cell volume didn't change, while in 0.25 *M* urea the cell exploded. To take into account the differing biological effects of solutions of the same osmolarity, we use the concept of **tonicity**. An **isotonic** solution has no final effect on cell volume; a solution that causes cells to swell at equilibrium is called a **hypotonic** solution; and a solution that causes cells to shrink at equilibrium is called a **hypertonic** solution. Thus, the 0.25 *M* sucrose solution was isotonic, and the 0.25 *M* urea solution was hypotonic. Note that an isotonic solution must have the same osmolarity as the fluid inside the cell, but that having the same osmolarity as the ICF does not guarantee that an external fluid is isotonic.

Time Course of Volume Changes

So far in the discussion of maintenance of cell volume, we have considered only the final, equilibrium effect of a solution on cell volume and have ignored any transient effects that may occur. To see such transient effects, consider what happens to the model cell immediately after it is placed in the solution used in Figure 2-4D, 0.25 *M* urea + 0.25 *M* sucrose. This is summarized in Figure 2-5. At the start, the osmolarity outside (0.5 Osm) is greater than the osmolarity inside (0.25 Osm), and water will initially leave the cell as it diffuses down its concentration gradient. Urea, however, begins to diffuse into the cell down its concentration gradient. Thus, the internal osmolarity begins to rise as a result of the increasing [urea]$_i$ and the loss of intracellular water. The leakage of water out of the cell slows down and finally ceases alto-

Figure 2-5

Time course of cell volume when the model cell is placed in the solution used in Figure 2-4D.

Time after placing cell in solution in Figure 2-4D

gether when $[P]_i + [urea]_i = 0.5\ M$, that is, at the point when internal and external osmolarities are equal. At this point, however, $[P]_i$ is higher than its initial value (0.25 M) because of the reduction in cell volume, and $[urea]_i$ is thus less than 0.25 M. Urea therefore continues to enter the cell to reach its own diffusion equilibrium, and the internal osmolarity rises above 0.5 Osm, so that water enters the cell and volume begins to increase. This situation continues until the final equilibrium state governed by Equations (2-4) and (2-6) is reached. What would you expect the time course of cell volume to be if the model cell were placed in an infinite volume of a solution of 0.5 M urea?

Summary

If animal cells are to survive, it is essential that they regulate the movement of water across the plasma membrane. Given that proteins and other organic constituents of the ICF cannot be allowed to cross the membrane, diffusion of water becomes a problem. Animal cells have solved this problem by excluding a compensating extracellular solute, sodium ions. Later we discuss in more detail exactly how they go about excluding Na^+.

Diffusion equilibrium is reached when internal and external concentrations are equal for all substances that can cross the membrane. For uncharged substances, such as those we considered in our examples so far, we do not have to consider the influence of electrical force on the equilibrium state. However, the solutes of the ICF and ECF of real cells bear a net electrical charge. In the next chapter, we consider what role electrical fields play in the movements of these charged substances across the membranes of animal cells.

Membrane Potential: Ionic Equilibrium

The central topics in Chapter 2 were the factors that influence the distribution of water across the plasma membrane and the strategies by which cells can attain osmotic equilibrium. For clarity, all the examples so far used only uncharged particles; however, a glance at Table 1-1 in Chapter 1 shows that all the solutes of both ICF and ECF are electrically charged. For charged particles, movement across the membrane is determined not only by diffusional force, but also by the electrical potential across the membrane. This chapter considers how cells can achieve equilibrium in the situation where both diffusional and electrical forces must be taken into account.

To illustrate the important principles that apply to ionic equilibrium, it is useful to work through a series of examples that are increasingly complex and increasingly similar to the situation in real animal cells. At the end of the series of examples, we will see how a model cell, with internal and external compositions like those given in Table 1-1, can be in electrical and chemical equilibrium. However, in the second part of this chapter, we will also see that this equilibrium model of the electrochemical state of cells does not apply to real animal cells, and that real cells must expend energy to maintain the distribution of ions across their plasma membranes.

Diffusion Potential

The names **cation** for positively charged particles and **anion** for negatively charged particles arise from the observation that dissolved positively charged particles accumulate around a wire connected to the negative pole, or cathode, of a battery and that dissolved negatively charged particles are attracted to a wire connected to the positive pole, or anode. The battery sets up a gradient of electrical potential (a **voltage** gradient) in the solution, and the movement of the ions in the solution is influenced by that voltage gradient. Thus, the distribution of ions in a solution depends on the presence of an electrical field in that solution. The other side of the coin is that a differential distribution of ions in a solution *gives rise to* a voltage gradient in the solution. As an example of how an electrical potential can arise from spatial differences in the distribution of ions, we consider the origin of **diffusion potentials**.

Diffusion potentials arise in the situation where two or more ions are moving down a concentration gradient. Examine the diagram in Figure 3-1, which shows a rigid container divided into two compartments by a porous barrier. In the left compartment we place a 0.1 M NaCl solution and in the right compartment a 1.0 M NaCl solution. The porous barrier allows Na^+, Cl^-, and water to cross, but because of the rigid walls the volume in the compartments is not free to change and water cannot move. Thus, osmotic factors can be neglected for the moment. However, both Na^+ and Cl^- will move down their concentration gradients from right to left until their concentrations are equal in both compartments. In aqueous solution, Na^+ and Cl^- do not move at the same rate; Cl^- is more mobile and moves from right to left more quickly than does Na^+. This is because ions dissolved in water carry with them a loosely associated "cloud" of water molecules, and Na^+ must drag along a larger cloud than Cl^-, causing it to move more slowly.

In Figure 3-1, then, the concentration of Cl^- on the left side will rise faster than the concentration of Na^+. In other words, there will be more negative than positive charges in the left compartment, and a voltmeter connected between the two sides would record a voltage difference, E, across the barrier, with the left compartment being negative with respect to the right compartment. This voltage difference is the diffusion potential. Notice that the electrical potential across the barrier tends to retard movement of Cl^- and speed up movement of Na^+ because the excess negative charges on the left repel Cl^- and attract Na^+. The diffusion potential will continue to build up until the electrical effect on the ions exactly counteracts the greater mobility of Cl^-, and the two ions cross the barrier at the same rate.

Another name for voltage is electromotive force. This name em-

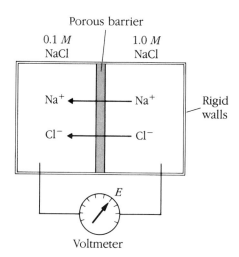

Porous barrier

0.1 *M*
NaCl

1.0 *M*
NaCl

$Na^+ \longleftarrow$ $\longleftarrow Na^+$

$Cl^- \longleftarrow$ $\longleftarrow Cl^-$

Rigid
walls

E

Voltmeter

Figure 3-1
Schematic diagram of an apparatus for measuring diffusion potential. The voltmeter is wired to measure the electrical voltage difference across the barrier separating the two salt solutions.

phasizes the fact that voltage is the driving force for the movement of electrical charges through space; without a voltage gradient there is no net movement of charged particles. Thus, voltage can be thought of as a pressure driving charges in a particular direction, just as the pressure in the water pipe drives water out through your tap when you open the valve. Unlike the pressure in a hydraulic system, however, a voltage gradient can move charges in two opposing directions, depending on the polarity of the charge. Thus, the negative pole of a battery simultaneously attracts positively charged particles and repels negatively charged particles.

Equilibrium Potential

The Nernst Equation

The diffusion potential example of Figure 3-1 does not describe an equilibrium condition, but rather a transient situation that occurs only as long as there is a net diffusion of ions across the barrier. Equilibrium would be achieved in Figure 3-1 only when $[Na^+]$ and $[Cl^-]$ are the same in compartments 1 and 2. At that point, there would be no concentrational force to support net diffusion of either Na^+ or Cl^- across the membrane and there would be no electrical potential across the barrier. Under what conditions might there be a steady electrical potential at equilibrium? To see this, consider a small modification to the previous example, shown in Figure 3-2. In the new example, everything is as before,

Figure 3-2

Schematic diagram of an apparatus for measuring the equilibrium, or Nernst, potential for a permeant ion. At equilibrium, there will be a steady electrical potential (the equilibrium potential) across the selectively permeable barrier separating the two salt solutions.

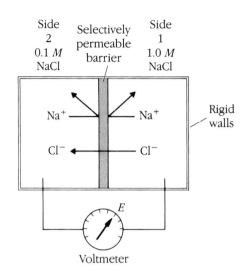

except that the barrier between the two compartments is selectively permeable to Cl^-: Na^+ cannot cross. Once again, we assume that the box has rigid walls so that we can neglect movement of water for the present.

The analysis of the situation in Figure 3-2 is similar to that of the diffusion potential example, except that now the "mobility" of Na^+ is reduced effectively to zero by the permeability characteristics of the barrier. Chloride ions will move down their concentration gradient from compartment 1 to compartment 2, but now no positive charges accompany them and negative charges will quickly build up in compartment 2. Thus, the voltmeter will record an electrical potential across the barrier, with side 2 being negative with respect to side 1. Because only Cl^- can cross the barrier, equilibrium will be reached when there is no further net movement of chloride across the barrier. This happens when the electrical force driving Cl^- out of compartment 2 exactly balances the concentrational force driving Cl^- out of compartment 1. Thus, at equilibrium a chloride ion moves from side 1 to side 2 down its concentration gradient for every chloride ion that moves from side 2 to side 1 down its electrical gradient. There will be no further change in $[Cl^-]$ in the two compartments, and no further change in the electrical potential, once this equilibrium has been reached.

Equilibrium for an ion is determined not only by concentrational forces but also by electrical forces. Movement of an ion across a cell membrane is determined both by the concentration gradient for that ion across the membrane and by the electrical potential difference across the membrane. We will use these ideas extensively in this book, so the remainder of this chapter examines how these principles apply in simple model situations and in real cells.

What would be the measured value of the voltage across the barrier at equilibrium in Figure 3-2? This is a quantitative question, and the answer is provided by Equation (3-1), which is called the **Nernst equation** after the physical chemist who derived it. The Nernst equation for Figure 3-2 can be written as follows:

$$E_{Cl} = (RT/ZF) \ln ([Cl^-]_1/[Cl^-]_2) \qquad (3\text{-}1)$$

Here, E_{Cl} is the voltage difference between sides 1 and 2 at equilibrium, R is the gas constant, T is the absolute temperature, Z is the valence of the ion in question (-1 for chloride), F is Faraday's constant, ln is the symbol for the natural, or base e, logarithm, and $[Cl^-]_1$ and $[Cl^-]_2$ are the chloride concentrations in compartments 1 and 2.

The value of electrical potential given by Equation (3-1) is called the **equilibrium potential**, or **Nernst potential**, for the ion in question. For example, in Figure 3-2 the permeant ion is chloride and the electrical potential, E_{Cl}, across the barrier is called the chloride equilibrium potential. If the barrier in Figure 3-2 allowed Na^+ to cross rather than Cl^-, Equation (3-1) would again apply, except that $[Na^+]_1$ and $[Na^+]_2$ would be used instead of $[Cl^-]$, and the valence would be $+1$ instead of -1. If sodium were the permeant ion, the resulting potential, E_{Na}, would be the sodium equilibrium potential. *The Nernst equation applies only to one ion at a time and only to ions that can cross the barrier.*

A derivation of Equation (3-1) is given in Appendix A. The Nernst equation comes from the realization that at equilibrium the total change in energy encountered by an ion in crossing the barrier must be zero. If the change in energy were not zero, there would be a net force driving the ion in one direction or the other, and the ion would not be at equilibrium. There are two important sources of energy change involved in crossing the barrier shown in Figure 3-2: the electrical field and the concentration gradient. Nernst arrived at his equation by setting the sum of the concentrational and electrical energy changes across the barrier to zero.

In biology, we usually work with a simplified form of Equation (3-1):

$$E_{Cl} = (58 \text{ mV}/Z) \log([Cl^-]_1/[Cl^-]_2) \qquad (3\text{-}2)$$

The simplification arises from converting from natural to base 10 logarithms, evaluating (RT/F) at standard room temperature (20°C), and expressing the result in millivolts (mV). That is where the constant 58 mV comes from in Equation (3-2). From the simplified Nernst equation, it can be seen that E_{Cl} in Figure 3-2 would be -58 mV. That is, in crossing the barrier from side 1 to side 2, we would encounter a potential change of 58 mV, with side 2 being negative with respect to side 1. This is as expected from the fact that chloride ions, and therefore negative charges, are accumulating on side 2. If the barrier were selectively permeable to Na^+ rather than Cl^-, the voltage across the barrier would be given by E_{Na}, which would be $+58$ mV given the values in Figure 3-2. What would be the equilibrium potential for chloride in Figure 3-2 if the concentration of NaCl was 1.0 M on both sides of the barrier? (Hint: In that case the concentration gradient would be zero.)

The Principle of Electrical Neutrality

In arriving at -58 mV for the chloride equilibrium potential in Figure 3-2, we used 1.0 M and 0.1 M for $[Cl^-]_1$ and $[Cl^-]_2$. These are the initial concentrations in the two compartments, even though in our qualitative analysis we said that Cl^- moved from compartment 1 to compartment 2, producing an excess of negative charge in compartment 2 and giving rise to the electrical potential. This would seem to suggest that $[Cl^-]$ changes from its initial value, invalidating our sample calculation. It is legitimate to use initial concentrations, however, because the increment in the electrical gradient caused by the movement of a single charged particle from compartment 1 to compartment 2 is very much larger than the decrement in concentration gradient resulting from movement of that same particle. Thus, *only a very small number of charges need accumulate in order to counter even a large concentration gradient.*

In Figure 3-2, for example, it is possible to calculate that if the volume of each compartment were 1 ml and if the barrier between compartments were 1 cm² of the same material found in cell membranes, it would require less than one-billionth of the chloride ions of side 1 to move to side 2 in order to reach the equilibrium potential of -58 mV. (The basis of this calculation is explained later.) Clearly, such a small change in concentration would produce an insignificant difference in the result calculated according to Equation (3-2), and we can safely ignore the movement of chloride necessary to achieve equilibrium.

This leads to an important principle that will be useful in the examples following in this chapter. This principle, called the **principle of electrical neutrality**, states that *under biological conditions the bulk concentration of cations within any compartment must be equal to the bulk concentration of anions in that compartment*. This is an acceptable approximation because the number of charges necessary to reach transmembrane potentials of the magnitude encountered in biology is insignificant compared with the total numbers of cations and anions in the intracellular and extracellular fluids.

The Cell Membrane as an Electrical Capacitor

This section explains how we were able to calculate the number of charges necessary to produce the equilibrium membrane potential of -58 mV in the preceding section. The calculation was made by treating the barrier between the two compartments as an electrical capacitor, which is a charge-storing device consisting of two conducting plates separated by an insulating barrier. In Figure 3-2, the two conducting plates are the salt solutions in the two compartments, and the barrier is the insulator. In a real cell, the ICF and ECF are the conductors, and the lipid bilayer of the plasma membrane is the insulating barrier. When a capacitor is hooked up to a battery as shown in Figure 3-3, the voltage of the battery causes electrons to be removed from one conducting plate and to accumulate on the other plate. This will continue until the resulting voltage gradient across the capacitor is equal to the voltage of the battery. Basic physics tells us that the amount of charge, q, stored on the capacitor at that time will be given by $q = CV$, where V is the voltage of the battery and C is the **capacitance** of the capacitor. A capacitor's capacitance is directly proportional to the area of the plates (bigger plates can store more charge) and inversely proportional to the distance separating the two plates. Capacitance also depends on the characteristics of the insulating material between the plates; in the case of cells, that insulating material is the lipid plasma membrane. The unit of capacitance is the farad (F): a 1 F capacitor can store 1 coulomb of charge when hooked up to a 1 V battery. Biological membranes, like the plasma membrane, have a capacitance of 10^{-6} F (that is, 1 microfarad, or μF) per square centimeter of membrane area.

If the barrier in Figure 3-2 were 1 cm^2 of cell membrane, it would therefore have a capacitance of 10^{-6} F. From $q = CV$, it fol-

Figure 3-3
When a battery is connected to a capacitor, charge accumulates on the capacitor until the voltage across the capacitor is equal to the voltage of the battery.

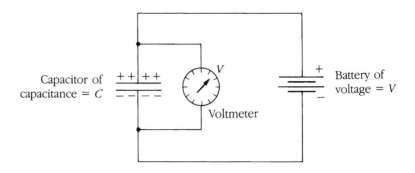

lows that an equilibrium potential of -58 mV would store 5.8×10^{-8} coulomb of charge on the barrier. Note that the charge on the membrane barrier in Figure 3-2 is carried by ions, not by electrons as in Figure 3-3. Thus, to know the total number of excess anions on side 2 of the barrier at equilibrium, we must convert from coulombs of charge to moles of ion. This can be done by dividing the number of coulombs on the barrier by Faraday's constant (approximately 10^5 coulombs per mole of monovalent ion), yielding 5.8×10^{-13} mole or about 3.5×10^{11} chloride ions moving from side 1 to side 2 in Figure 3-2. If the volume of each compartment were 1 ml, then side 2 would contain about 6×10^{20} chloride and sodium ions. This leads to the conclusion stated in the previous section that less than one-billionth of the chloride ions in side 1 cross to side 2 to produce the equilibrium voltage across the barrier.

Incorporating Osmotic Balance

The example shown in Figure 3-2 illustrates how ionic equilibrium can be reached and how the Nernst equation can be used to calculate the value of the membrane potential at equilibrium. However, the simple situation in the example is not very similar to the situation in real animal cells. For one thing, animal cells are not enclosed in a box with rigid walls, and thus osmotic balance must be taken into account. An example of how equilibrium can be reached when water balance must be considered is shown in Figure 3-4A. In this example the rigid walls are removed, so that osmotic balance must be achieved in order to reach equilibrium. In addition, an impermeant intracellular solute, P, has been added. For now, P has no charge; the effect of adding a charge on the intracellular organic solute is considered later in this chapter.

In Figure 3-4A, it is assumed that the model cell contains 50

(A)

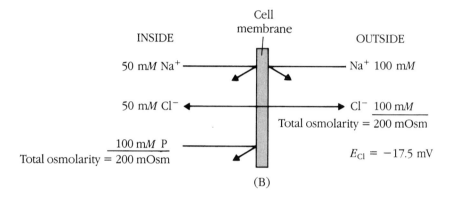

(B)

Figure 3-4
A model cell in which both osmotic and electrical factors must be considered at equilibrium.

mM Na$^+$ and 100 mM P. What must the concentrations of the other intracellular and extracellular solutes be in order for the model cell to be at equilibrium? The principle of electrical neutrality tells us that for practical purposes, the concentrations of cations and anions within any compartment are equal. Thus, because P is assumed to have no charge, [Cl$^-$]$_i$ = [Na$^+$]$_i$ = 50 mM. For osmotic balance, the external osmolarity must equal the internal osmolarity, which is 200 mOsm. The principle of electrical neutrality again requires that [Na$^+$]$_o$ = [Cl$^-$]$_o$. This requirement, together with the requirement for osmotic balance, can be satisfied if [Na$^+$]$_o$ = [Cl$^-$]$_o$ = 100 mM. The model cell of Figure 3-4A can therefore be at equilibrium if the concentrations of intracellular and extracellular solutes are as shown in Figure 3-4B. At this equilibrium, the electrical potential across the membrane of the model cell (the membrane potential, E_m) would be given by the Nernst equation for chloride:

$$E_m = E_{Cl} = -58 \text{ mV log } ([Cl^-]_o/[Cl^-]_i) = -17.5 \text{ mV}$$

Donnan Equilibrium

The example of Figure 3-4B shows how we could construct a model cell that is simultaneously at osmotic and ionic equilibrium. However, the situation in Figure 3-4B is not very much like that in real animal cells. A major difference is that the principal internal cation in real cells is K^+, not Na^+. Also, there is some potassium in the ECF, and the cell membrane is permeable to K^+ as well as Cl^-. In this situation, there are two ions that can cross the membrane: K^+ and Cl^-. If equilibrium is to be reached, the electrical potential across the cell membrane must exactly balance the concentration gradients for both K^+ and Cl^-. Because the membrane potential can have only one value, this equilibrium condition will be satisfied only when the equilibrium potentials for Cl^- and K^+ are equal. In equation form, this condition can be written as follows:

$$E_K = 58 \text{ mV log } ([K^+]_o/[K^+]_i) = E_{Cl} = -58 \text{ mV log } ([Cl^-]_o/[Cl^-]_i)$$

Here, the minus sign on the far right arises from the fact that the valence of chloride is -1. Canceling 58 mV from the above relation leaves

$$\log ([K^+]_o/[K^+]_i) = -\log ([Cl^-]_o/[Cl^-]_i) \qquad (3\text{-}3)$$

The minus sign on the right side can be moved inside the parentheses of the logarithm to yield $\log([Cl^-]_i/[Cl^-]_o)$. Thus, equilibrium will be reached when

$$([K^+]_o/[K^+]_i) = ([Cl^-]_i/[Cl^-]_o) \qquad (3\text{-}4)$$

This equilibrium condition is called the **Donnan** or **Gibbs-Donnan equilibrium**, and it specifies the conditions that must be met if two ions that can cross a cell membrane are simultaneously to be at equilibrium across that membrane. Equation (3-4) is usually written in a slightly rearranged form as the product of concentrations:

$$[K^+]_o[Cl^-]_o = [K^+]_i[Cl^-]_i \qquad (3\text{-}5)$$

In words, for a Donnan equilibrium to hold, the product of the concentrations of the permeant ions outside the cell must be equal

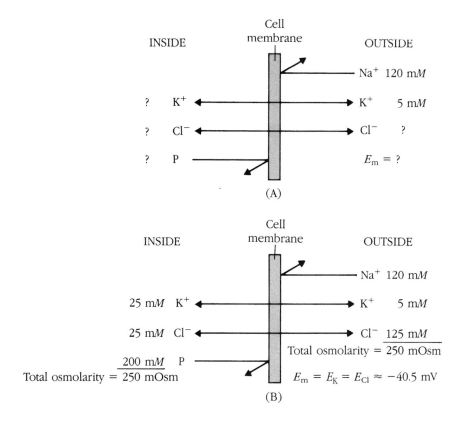

Figure 3-5
An example of a model cell at
Donnan equilibrium. The cell
membrane is permeable to both
potassium and chloride.

to the product of the concentrations of those two ions inside the cell.

To see how the Donnan equilibrium might apply in an animal cell, consider the example shown in Figure 3-5A. Here a model cell containing K^+, Cl^-, and P is placed in ECF containing Na^+, K^+, and Cl^-. As an exercise, we will calculate the values of all concentrations at equilibrium assuming that $[Na^+]_o$ is 120 mM and $[K^+]_o$ is 5 mM. From the principal of electrical neutrality, $[Cl^-]_o$ must be 125 mM. Also, because P is assumed for the present to be uncharged, the principle of electrical neutrality requires that $[K^+]_i$ must equal $[Cl^-]_i$. Because two ions—K^+ and Cl^-—can cross the membrane, the defining relation for a Donnan equilibrium shown in Equation (3-5) must be obeyed. Thus, if the model cell of Figure 3-5A is to be at equilibrium, $[K^+]_i[Cl^-]_i$ must equal $[K^+]_o[Cl^-]_o$, which is 5×125, or 625 mM^2. Because $[K^+]_i = [Cl^-]_i$, the Donnan condition reduces to $[K^+]_i^2 = 625$ mM^2; thus, $[K^+]_i$ and $[Cl^-]_i$ must be 25 mM at equilibrium. For osmotic balance, the internal osmolarity must equal the external osmolarity, which is

250 mOsm. This requires that $[P]_i$ must be 200 mM for the model cell to be at equilibrium. The results of this example are summarized in Figure 3-5B, which represents a model cell at equilibrium. What would be the membrane potential of this equilibrated model cell? The Nernst equation—Equation (3-2)—tells us that the membrane potential for a cell at equilibrium with $[K^+]_o = 5$ mM and $[K^+]_i = 25$ mM is about -40.5 mV, inside negative. You should satisfy yourself that the Nernst equation for chloride yields the same value for membrane potential.

A Model Cell That Looks Like a Real Animal Cell

The model cell of Figure 3-5B still lacks many features of real animal cells. For instance, as Table 1-1 shows, the internal organic molecules are charged, and this charge must be considered in the balance between cations and anions required by the principle of electrical neutrality. Recall that the category of internal anions, A^-, actually represents a diverse group of molecules, including proteins, charged amino acids, and sulfate and phosphate ions. Some of these bear a single negative charge, others bear two charges, and some even three net negative charges. Taken as a group, however, the average charge per molecule is slightly greater than -1.2. Thus, the internal impermeant anions can be represented as $A^{1.2-}$.

In addition, the model cell of Figure 3-5B lacks Na^+ inside the cell, while real ICF does contain a small amount of sodium. Addition of these complicating factors leads to the model cell of Figure 3-6A, which now contains all the constituents shown in Table 1-1. If the cell of Figure 3-6A is to be at equilibrium, what concentrations of the various ions in ECF and ICF would be required, and what would be the transmembrane potential? To begin, we take some values from Table 1-1 and determine what the remaining parameters must be for the cell to be at equilibrium. Assume that $[K^+]_o = 5$ mM, $[Na^+]_o = 120$ mM, $[Cl^-]_i = 5$ mM, and $[A^{1.2-}]_i = 108$ mM. (Actually, it is not necessary to assume the concentration of A; it could be calculated from the other parameters. For mathematical simplicity, however, we will assume that it is known from the start.) Because Cl^- is the sole external anion, the principle of electrical neutrality requires that $[Cl^-]_o$ be 125 mM. Both K^+ and Cl^- can cross the membrane, so that the conditions for a Donnan

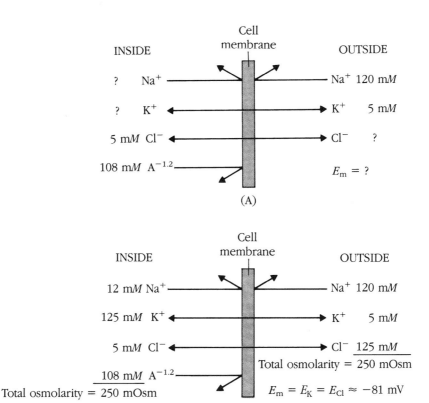

Figure 3-6

An example of a realistic model cell that is at both electrical and osmotic equilibrium. The compositions of ECF and ICF for this equilibrated model cell are the same as for a typical mammalian cell (see Table 1-1).

equilibrium—Equation (3-5)—must be satisfied. This requires that $[K^+]_i = 125$ mM. The equilibrated value of $[Na^+]_i$ can then be obtained from the requirements for osmotic balance; $[Na^+]_i$ must be 12 mM if internal and external osmolarities are to be equal. From the Nernst equation for either Cl^- or K^+, the membrane potential at equilibrium can be determined to be about −81 mV.

The equilibrium values for this model cell are shown in Figure 3-6B. Note that the concentrations of all intracellular and extracellular solutes are the same for the model cell and for real mammalian cells (see Table 1-1). The values in Figure 3-6B were arrived at by assuming that the cell was in equilibrium, and this implies that the real cell, which has the same ECF and ICF, is also at equilibrium. Thus, the model cell, and by extension the real cell, will remain in the state summarized in Figure 3-6B without expending any metabolic energy at all. From this viewpoint, the animal cell is a beautiful example of efficiency, existing at perfect equilibrium, both ionic and osmotic, in harmony with its electrochemical environment. The problem, however, is that the model cell is not an accurate representation of the situation in real animal cells: *Real cells are not at equilibrium and must expend metabolic energy to maintain the status quo.*

The Sodium Pump

For some time, the model in Figure 3-6B was thought to be an accurate description of real animal cells. The difficulty with this scheme arose when it became apparent that real cells are permeable to sodium, while the model cell is assumed to be impermeable to sodium. Permeability to sodium, however, would be catastrophic for the model cell. If sodium can cross the membrane, then all extracellular solutes can cross the membrane. Recall from Chapter 2, however, what happens to cells that are placed in ECF containing only permeant solutes (like the urea example in Figure 2-4C): The cell swells and bursts. The cornerstone of the strategy employed by animal cells to achieve osmotic balance is that the cell membrane must exclude an extracellular solute to balance the impermeant organic solutes inside the cell. Sodium ions played that role for the model cell of Figure 3-6B.

How can the permeability of the plasma membrane to sodium be reconciled with the requirement for osmotic balance? An answer to this question was suggested by experiments that demonstrated the sodium permeability of the cell membrane in the first place. In these experiments, red blood cells were incubated in an external medium containing radioactive sodium ions. When the cells were removed from the radioactive medium and washed thoroughly, it was found that they remained radioactive, indicating that the cells had taken up some of the radioactive sodium. This showed that the plasma membrane was permeable to sodium. In addition, it was found that the radioactive cells slowly lost their radioactive sodium when incubated in normal ECF. This latter observation was surprising because both the concentration gradient and the electrical gradient for sodium are directed inward; neither would tend to move sodium out of the cell. Further, the rate of this loss of radioactive sodium from the cell interior was slowed dramatically by cooling the cells, indicating that a source of energy other than simple diffusion was being tapped to actively "pump" sodium out of the cell against its concentrational and electrical gradients. It turns out that this energy source is metabolic energy in the form of the high-energy phosphate compound adenosine triphosphate (ATP).

This active pumping of sodium out of the cell effectively prevents sodium from accumulating intracellularly as it leaks in down its concentration and electrical gradients. Thus, even though sodium can cross the membrane, it is actively extruded at a rate sufficiently high to counterbalance the inward leak. The net result is that *sodium behaves osmotically as though it cannot cross the membrane*. Note however that this mechanism is fundamentally different from the situation in the model cell of Figure 3-6B. The model was in *equilibrium* and required no energy input to maintain itself. In contrast, real animal cells are in a finely balanced *steady state*, in which there is no net movement of ions across the cell membrane, but which requires the expenditure of metabolic energy.

Metabolic inhibitors, such as cyanide and dinitrophenol, prevent the pumping of sodium out of the cell and cause cells to gain sodium and swell. If ATP is added, the pump can operate once again and the accumulated sodium will be extruded. Similarly, other manipulations that reduce the rate of ATP production, like cooling, cause sodium accumulation and increased cell volume. Experiments of this type demonstrated the role of ATP in the active extrusion of sodium and the maintenance of cell volume. The mechanism of the sodium pump has been studied biochemically. The pump itself is a particular kind of membrane-associated protein molecule that can bind both sodium ions and ATP at the intracellular face of the membrane. The protein then acts as an enzyme to cleave one of the high-energy phosphate bonds of the ATP molecule, using the released energy to drive the bound sodium out across the membrane by a process that is not yet completely understood.

The action of the sodium pump also requires potassium ions in the ECF. Binding of K^+ to a part of the protein on the outer surface of the cell membrane is required for the protein to return to the configuration in which it can again bind another ATP and sodium ions at the inner surface of the membrane. The potassium bound on the outside is released again on the inside of the cell, so that the protein molecule acts as a bidirectional pump carrying sodium out across the membrane and potassium in. Thus, the sodium pump is more correctly referred to as the sodium-potassium pump, and can be thought of as a shuttle carrying Na^+ out across the membrane, releasing it in the ECF, then carrying K^+ in across the membrane and releasing it in the ICF. Because the pump molecule splits ATP and binds both sodium and potassium ions, biochemists refer to this membrane-associated enzyme as a Na^+/K^+ ATPase.

Summary

The movement of charged substances across the plasma membrane is governed not only by the concentration gradient across the membrane but also by the electrical potential across the membrane. Equilibrium for an ion across the membrane is reached when the electrical gradient exactly balances the concentration gradient for that ion. The equation that expresses this equilibrium condition quantitatively is the Nernst equation, which gives the value of membrane potential that will exactly balance a given concentration gradient.

If more than one ion can cross the cell membrane, both can be at equilibrium only if the Nernst, or equilibrium, potentials for both ions are the same. This requirement leads to the defining properties of the Donnan, or Gibbs-Donnan, equilibrium, which applies simultaneously to two permeant ions. By working through a series of examples, we saw how it is possible to build a model cell that is at equilibrium and that has ICF, ECF, and membrane potential like that of real animal cells.

Real cells, however, were found to be permeable to sodium ions. This removed an important cornerstone of the equilibrated model cell, and forced a change in viewpoint about the relation between animal cells and their environment. Real cells must expend metabolic energy, in the form of ATP, in order to "pump" sodium out against its concentration and electrical gradients and thus to maintain osmotic balance. In the next chapter, we consider what effect the sodium permeability of the plasma membrane might have on the electrical membrane potential. We show how the membrane potential depends not only on the concentrations of ions on the two sides of the membrane, as in the Nernst equation, but also on the relative permeability of the membrane to those ions.

4

Membrane Potential: Ionic Steady State

In the last chapter, we learned that it is possible for two permeant ions to be at equilibrium across a cell membrane simultaneously. This Donnan equilibrium required that the membrane potential be equal to the Nernst potentials for the two ions. However, we also saw that real animal cells are permeable to sodium and thus that there are three major ions—potassium, chloride, and sodium—that can cross the plasma membrane. This chapter is concerned with the effect of sodium permeability on membrane potential and with the quantitative relation between ionic permeabilities and concentrations on the one hand and electrical membrane potential on the other.

Equilibrium Potentials for Sodium, Potassium, and Chloride

If the permeability of the cell membrane to sodium is not zero, then the resting membrane potential of the cell must have a contribution from Na^+ as well as from K^+ and Cl^-. This is true even though the sodium pump eventually removes any sodium that leaks into the cell. There are two reasons for this. First, recall that the electrical force per particle is much stronger than the concentrational force per particle; therefore, even a tiny trickle of sodium that would cause a negligible change in internal concentration could produce large changes in membrane potential. Because the sodium pump responds only to changes in the bulk concentration of sodium inside the cell, it cannot detect and respond to the

39

tiny changes that would occur for even large changes in membrane potential. Second, even though sodium that leaks in is eventually pumped out, the efflux of sodium through the pump is coupled with an influx of potassium. Thus, there is a net transfer of positive charge into the cell associated with leakage of sodium.

Application of the Nernst equation to the concentrations of sodium, potassium, and chloride in the ICF and ECF of a typical mammalian cell (see Table 1-1) shows that the membrane potential cannot possibly be simultaneously at the equilibrium potentials of all three ions. As we calculated in Chapter 3, $E_K = E_{Cl} =$ about -80 mV (actually a bit greater than -81 mV, given the values in Table 1-1). But with $[Na^+]_o = 120$ mM and $[Na^+]_i = 12$ mM, E_{Na} would be $+58$ mV. The membrane potential, E_m, cannot simultaneously be at -80 mV and $+58$ mV. The actual value of membrane potential will fall somewhere between these two extreme values. If the sodium permeability of the membrane were in fact zero, E_m would be determined solely by E_K and E_{Cl} and would be -80 mV. Conversely, if chloride and potassium permeability were zero, E_m would be determined only by sodium and would lie at E_{Na}, $+58$ mV. Because the permeabilities of all three ions are not zero, there will be a struggle between Na^+ on the one hand, tending to make E_m equal $+58$ mV, and K^+ and Cl^- on the other, tending to make E_m equal -80 mV. Two factors determine where E_m will actually fall: (1) ion concentrations, which determine the equilibrium potentials for the ions; and (2) relative ion permeabilities, which determine the relative importance of a particular ion in governing where E_m lies. Before we express these relations quantitatively, it is useful to consider the mechanism of ionic permeability in more detail.

Ionic Channels in the Plasma Membrane

The permeability of a membrane to a particular ion is a measure of the ease with which that ion can cross the membrane. It is a property of the membrane itself. Recall that ions cannot cross membranes through the lipid portion of the membrane; they must cross through aqueous pores or channels in the membrane. Thus, the ionic permeability of a membrane is determined by the properties of the ionic pores or channels in that membrane. The total permeability of a membrane to a particular ion is governed by the total number of membrane channels that allow that ion to cross and by the ease with which the ion can go through a single channel. Ionic channels are protein molecules that are associated with the membrane, and thus an important function of membrane proteins is the regulation of ionic permeability of the cell membrane. In later chapters, we discuss how specialized channels modulate ionic permeability in response to chemical or electrical signals and the role of such changes in permeability in the processing of signals in the nervous system.

Not all membrane channels allow all ions to cross with equal ease. Some channels allow only cations through, and others only anions. Some channels are even more selective, allowing only K^+ through but not Na^+, or vice versa. Thus, it is possible for a membrane to have very different permeabilities to different ions, depending on the number of channels for each ion.

Membrane Potential and Ionic Permeability

As an example of how the actual value of membrane potential depends on the relative permeabilities of the competing ions, consider the situation illustrated in Figure 4-1. This model cell is much more permeable to K^+ than to Na^+. In other words, there are many channels that allow K^+ to cross the membrane but only a few that allow Na^+ to cross. Imagine that initially we connect the cell to an apparatus that artificially maintains the resting membrane potential at E_K, so that $E_m = E_K = -80$ mV. (This can be accomplished experimentally using a voltage-clamp apparatus, as described in Chapter 6.) What will happen to E_m when we switch off the apparatus and allow E_m to take on any value it wishes? In order to determine what will happen, it is necessary to keep in mind one important principle: *If the membrane potential is not equal to the equilibrium potential for an ion, that ion will move across the membrane in such a way as to force E_m toward the equilibrium potential for that ion.* For example, Figure 4-2 illustrates the movement of K^+ across a cell membrane in response to changes in E_m. In this example, a cell is connected to an apparatus that allows us to set the membrane potential to any value we choose. Initially, we set E_m to E_K. Recall from Chapter 3 that when $E_m = E_K$ there is a balance between the electrical force driving K^+ into the cell and the concentrational force driving K^+ out of the

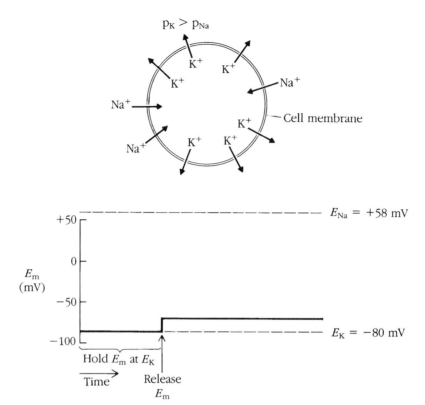

Figure 4-1
The resting membrane potential of a cell that is more permeable to potassium than to sodium. At the upward arrow, an apparatus that artificially holds the membrane potential at E_K abruptly switched off, and E_m is allowed to seek its own resting level.

cell. At time *a*, however, we suddenly make the interior of the cell less negative, reducing the electrical potential across the cell membrane and therefore decreasing the electrical force driving K^+ into the cell. Such a reduction in the electrical potential across the membrane is called a depolarization of the membrane. The electrical force will then be weaker than the oppositely directed concentrational force, and there will be a net movement of K^+ out of the cell. Note that this movement is in the proper direction to make E_m move back toward E_K, that is, to make the interior of the cell more negative because of the efflux of positive charge. At time *b*, we suddenly make E_m more negative than E_K; that is, we hyperpolarize the membrane. Now the electrical force will be stronger than the concentrational force and there will be a net movement of K^+ into the cell. Again, this is in the proper direction to make E_m move toward E_K, in this case by adding positive charge to the interior of the cell.

Return now to Figure 4-1. We would expect that Na^+, which

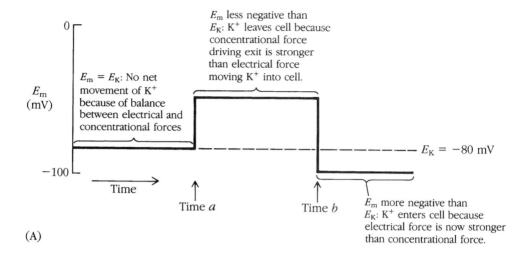

E_m less negative than
E_K: K⁺ leaves cell because
concentrational force
driving exit is stronger
than electrical force
moving K⁺ into cell.

$E_m = E_K$: No net
movement of K⁺
because of balance
between electrical and
concentrational forces

E_m
(mV)

$E_K = -80$ mV

-100

Time

Time *a*

Time *b*

E_m more negative than
E_K: K⁺ enters cell because
electrical force is now stronger
than concentrational force.

(A)

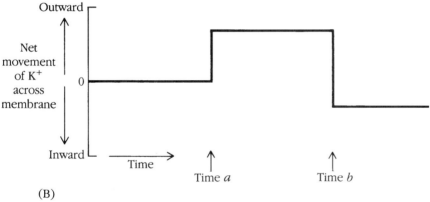

Outward

Net
movement
of K⁺
across
membrane

0

Inward

Time

Time *a*

Time *b*

(B)

Figure 4-2

Effect of changes in membrane potential on the movement of potassium ions across the plasma membrane. When the membrane potential is artificially manipulated (A), potassium ions move across the membrane in a direction governed by the difference between E_m and E_K (B).

has an equilibrium potential of +58 mV, will enter the cell. That is, Na⁺ will bring positive charge into the cell, and when we switch off the apparatus forcing E_m to remain at E_K, this influx of sodium ions will cause the membrane potential to become more positive (that is, move toward E_{Na}). As E_m moves toward E_{Na}, however, it will no longer be equal to E_K, and K⁺ will move out of the cell in response to the resulting imbalance between the potassium concentrational force and electrical force. Thus, there will be a struggle between K⁺ efflux forcing E_m toward E_K and Na⁺ influx forcing E_m toward E_{Na}. Because K⁺ permeability is much higher than Na⁺ permeability, potassium ions can move out readily to counteract the electrical effect of the trickle of sodium ions

Figure 4-3
The resting membrane potential of a cell that is more permeable to sodium than to potassium. As in Figure 4-1, an apparatus holding E_m at E_K is abruptly turned off at the upward arrow.

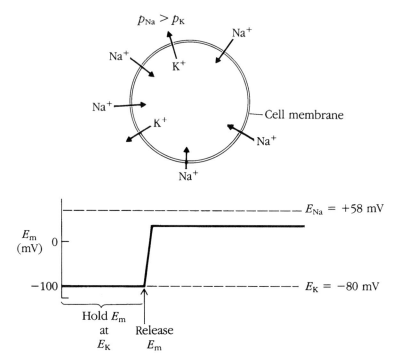

into the cell. Thus, in this situation, the balance between the movement of Na^+ into the cell and the exit of K^+ from the cell would be struck relatively close to E_K.

Figure 4-3 shows a different situation. In this case, everything is as before except that the sodium permeability is much greater than the potassium permeability. That is, there are more channels that allow Na^+ across than allow K^+ across. Once again, we start with $E_m = E_K = -80$ mV and then allow E_m to seek its own value. Sodium, with $E_{Na} = +58$ mV, enters the cell down its electrical and concentration gradients. The resulting accumulation of positive charge again causes the cell to depolarize, as before. Now, however, potassium cannot move out as readily as sodium can move in, and the influx of sodium will not be balanced as readily by an efflux of potassium. Thus, E_m will move farther from E_K and will reach a steady value closer to E_{Na} than to E_K.

The point of the previous two examples is that the value of membrane potential will be governed by the relative permeabilities of the permeant ions. *If a cell membrane is highly permeable to an ion, that ion can respond readily to deviations away from its equilibrium potential and E_m will tend to be near that equilibrium potential.*

The Goldman Equation

The examples discussed so far concerned the qualitative relation between membrane potential and relative ionic permeabilities. The equation that gives the quantitative relation between E_m on the one hand and ion concentrations and permeabilities on the other is the **Goldman equation**, which is also called the **constant-field equation.** For a cell that is permeable to potassium, sodium and chloride, the Goldman equation can be written as follows:

$$E_m = \frac{RT}{F} \ln\left(\frac{p_K[K^+]_o + p_{Na}[Na^+]_o + p_{Cl}[Cl^-]_i}{p_K[K^+]_i + p_{Na}[Na^+]_i + p_{Cl}[Cl^-]_o} \right) \quad (4\text{-}1)$$

This equation is similar to the Nernst equation (see Chapter 3), except that it simultaneously takes into account the contributions of all permeant ions. Some information about the derivation of the Goldman equation can be found in Appendix B. Note that the concentration of each ion on the right side of the equation is scaled according to its permeability, p. Thus, if the cell is highly permeable to potassium, for example, the potassium term on the right will dominate and E_m will be near the Nernst potential for potassium. Note also that if p_{Na} and p_{Cl} were zero, the Goldman equation would reduce to the Nernst equation for potassium, and E_m would be exactly equal to E_K, as we would expect if the only permeant ion were potassium.

Because it is easier to measure relative ion permeabilities than it is to measure absolute permeabilities, the Goldman equation is often written in a slightly different form:

$$E_m = 58\,\text{mV} \log\left(\frac{[K^+]_o + b[Na^+]_o + c[Cl^-]_i}{[K^+]_i + b[Na^+]_i + c[Cl^-]_o} \right) \quad (4\text{-}2)$$

In this case, the permeabilities have been expressed relative to the permeability of the membrane to potassium. Thus, $b = p_{Na}/p_K$, and $c = p_{Cl}/p_K$. We have also evaluated RT/F at room temperature, converted from ln to log, and expressed the result in millivolts.

For most nerve cells, the Goldman equation can be simplified even further: The chloride term on the right can be dropped altogether. This approximation is valid because the contribution of chloride to the resting membrane potential is insignificant in most nerve cells. In this case, the Goldman equation becomes

$$E_m = 58\,\text{mV} \log\left(\frac{[K^+]_o + b[Na^+]_o}{[K^+]_i + b[Na^+]_i}\right) \tag{4-3}$$

This is the form typically encountered in neurophysiology. In nerve cells, the ratio of sodium to potassium permeability, b, is commonly about 0.02, although this value may vary somewhat from one type of cell to another. That is, p_K is about 50 times higher than p_{Na}. Thus, Equation (4-3) tells us that E_m would be about −71 mV for a cell with $[K^+]_i = 125$ mM, $[K^+]_o = 5$ mM, $[Na^+]_i = 12$ mM, $[Na^+]_o = 120$ mM, and $b = 0.02$. What would E_m be for the same cell if b were 1.0 (that is, if $p_{Na} = p_K$) instead of 0.02?

The Goldman equation tells us quantitatively what we would expect qualitatively. If p_K is 50 times higher than p_{Na}, we would expect E_m to be nearer to E_K than to E_{Na}. Indeed, Equation (4-3) yields $E_m = −71$ mV, which is much nearer to E_K (−80 mV) than to E_{Na} (+58 mV). The difference between E_m and E_K reflects the steady influx of sodium ions carrying positive charge into the cell and maintaining a depolarization from E_K.

The applicability of the Goldman equation to a real cell can be tested experimentally by varying the concentration of potassium in the ECF and measuring the resulting changes in membrane potential. If membrane potential were determined solely by the distribution of potassium ions across the cell membrane—that is, if the factor b in Equation (4-3) were zero—we know that E_m would be determined by the potassium equilibrium potential. In this situation, a plot of measured membrane potential against log $[K^+]_o$ would yield a straight line with a slope of 58 mV per tenfold change in $[K^+]_o$. This straight line would merely be a plot of the E_m calculated from the Nernst equation at different values for external potassium concentration, and it is shown by the dashed line in Figure 4-4. Look, however, at the actual data from a real experiment in Figure 4-4. These data are the measured values of E_m of a nerve fiber observed at a number of different external potassium concentrations. The data do not follow the line expected from the Nernst equation, but instead fall along the solid line. That line was drawn according to the form of the Goldman equation given in Equation (4-3), and this experiment demonstrates that the real value of the membrane potential in the nerve fiber is determined jointly by potassium and sodium ions. Experiments of this type by Hodgkin and Katz in 1949 first demonstrated the role of sodium ions in the resting membrane potential of real cells.

Equation (4-3) is a reasonable approximation to Equation (4-2)

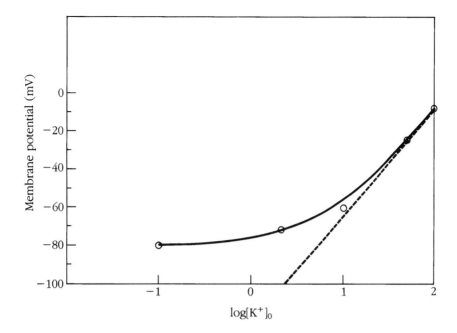

Figure 4-4
Experimentally determined
relation between external
potassium concentration and
resting membrane potential of
an axon in the spinal cord of the
lamprey. The circles represent
the measured values of
membrane potential at five
different values of $[K^+]_o$. The
dashed line gives the potassium
equilibrium potential calculated
from the Nernst equation. The
solid line shows the prediction
from the Goldman equation with
internal and external sodium and
potassium concentrations
appropriate for the lamprey
nervous system.

only if p_{Cl}/p_K is negligible. To determine whether it is valid to ignore the contribution of chloride—that is, to use Equation (4-3)—experiments like that summarized in Figure 4-4 can be performed in which the concentration of chloride in the ECF, rather than the concentration of potassium, is varied. When that was done on the type of nerve cell used in the experiment of Figure 4-4, it was found that a tenfold reduction of $[Cl^-]_o$ caused only a 2 mV change in the resting membrane potential. Thus, for that type of cell, membrane potential is relatively unaffected by chloride concentration, and Equation (4-3) is valid. This is also true for other nerve cells. It is important to emphasize, however, that the membranes of other kinds of cells, such as muscle cells, have larger chloride permeability; therefore, the membrane potential of those cells more strongly depends on the external chloride concentration. This was demonstrated experimentally for muscle cells by Hodgkin and Horowicz.

Ionic Steady State

The Goldman equation represents the actual situation in animal cells. The membrane potential of the cell takes on a steady value that reflects a fine balance between competing influences. It is important to keep in mind that neither sodium ions nor potassium ions are at equilibrium at that steady value of potential: Sodium ions are continually leaking into the cell and potassium ions are continually leaking out. If this were allowed to continue, the concentration gradients for sodium and potassium would eventually run down and the membrane potential would decline to zero as the ionic gradients collapsed. It is like a flashlight that has been left on: The batteries slowly discharge.

To prevent the intracellular accumulation of sodium and loss of potassium, the cell must expend energy to restore the ionic gradients. Here again is an important role for the sodium pump. Metabolic energy stored in ATP is used to extrude the sodium that leaks in and to regain the potassium that was lost. In this way, the batteries are recharged using metabolic energy. Viewed in this light, we can see that the steady membrane potential of a cell represents chemical energy that has been converted into a different form and stored in the ionic gradients across the cell membrane. In Part II of this book, beginning with Chapter 5, we will see how some cells, most notably the cells that make up the nervous system, are able to tap this stored energy to generate signals that can carry information and allow animals to move about and function in their environment.

The Chloride Pump

Because the resting membrane potential of a cell is not at either the sodium or the potassium equilibrium potential, there is a continuous net flux of sodium across the membrane. As we have just seen, metabolic energy must be expended in order to maintain the ionic gradients for sodium and potassium. What about chloride? The equilibrium potential for chloride, given the internal and external concentrations shown in Table 1-1, would be about −80 mV, but the resting membrane potential is about −71 mV. Thus, we would expect that there would be a steady influx of chloride into the cell because of this imbalance between the electrical and concentration gradients for chloride. Eventually, this influx would raise the internal chloride concentration to the point where the new chloride equilibrium potential would be −71 mV, the same as the resting membrane potential. At that point the concentration gradient for chloride would be reduced sufficiently to come into balance with the resting membrane potential. We can calculate from the Nernst equation that chloride would have to rise to about 7.5 mM from its usual 5 mM in order for this new equilibrium state to be established.

In some cells, this does appear to happen: Chloride reaches a new equilibrium governed by the resting membrane potential of the cell. (The cell would also gain the same small amount of potassium; because there is so much potassium inside, a change in potassium concentration by a few millimolar makes very little change in the potassium equilibrium potential, however.) In other cells, however, the chloride equilibrium potential remains different from the resting membrane potential, just as the sodium and potassium equilibrium potentials remain different from E_m. The only way this nonequilibrium condition can be maintained is by expending energy to keep the internal chloride constant—that is, there must also be a chloride pump similar in function to the sodium–potassium pump. In most cells, the chloride pump moves chloride ions out of the cell, so that the chloride equilibrium potential remains more negative than the resting membrane potential. In a few cases, however, an inwardly directed chloride pump has been discovered. Less is known about the molecular machinery of the chloride pump than of the sodium–potassium pump. It is thought to involve an ATPase in some instances, so that the energy released by hydrolysis of ATP is the immediate driving energy for the pumping. In other cases, the pump may use energy stored in gradients of other ions to drive the movement of chloride.

Electrical Current and the Movement of Ions Across Membranes

An electrical current is the movement of charge through space. In a wire like that carrying electricity in your house, the electrical current is a flow of electrons; in a solution of ions, however, a flow of current is carried by movement of ions. That is, in a solution, the charges that move during an electrical current flow are the charges on the ions in solution. Thus, the movement of ions through space—such as from the outside of a cell to the inside of a cell—constitutes an electrical current, just as the movement of electrons through a wire constitutes an electrical current.

By thinking of ion flows as electrical currents, we can get a different perspective on the factors governing the steady-state membrane potential of cells. We have seen that at the steady-state value of membrane potential, there is a steady influx of sodium ions into the cell and a steady efflux of potassium ions out of the cell. This means that there is a steady electrical current, carried by sodium ions, flowing across the cell membrane in one direction and another current, carried by potassium ions, flowing across the membrane in the opposite direction. By convention, it is assumed that electrical current flows from the plus to the minus terminal of a battery; that is, we talk about currents in a wire as though the current is carried by positive charges. By extension, this convention means that the sodium current is an *inward* membrane current (the transfer of positive charge from the outside to the inside of the membrane), and the potassium current is an *outward* membrane current.

As we saw in our earlier discussion of the Goldman equation, a steady value of membrane potential will be achieved when the influx of sodium is exactly balanced by the efflux of potassium. In electrical terms, this means that in the steady state the sodium current, i_{Na}, is equal and opposite to the potassium current, i_K. In equation form, this can be written as follows:

$$i_K + i_{Na} = 0 \qquad (4\text{-}4)$$

Thus, at the steady state the net membrane current is zero. This makes electrical sense, if we keep in mind that the cell membrane can be treated as an electrical capacitor (see Chapter 3). If the sum of i_{Na} and i_K were not zero, there would be a net flow of current across the membrane. Thus, there would be a movement of charge onto (or from) the membrane capacitor. Any such movement of charge would change the voltage across the capacitor (the membrane potential); that is, from the relation $q = CV$, if q changes and C remains constant, then V must of necessity change. Equation (4-4), then, is a requirement of the steady-state condition; if the equation is not true, the membrane potential cannot be at a steady level.

In cells in which there is an appreciable flow of chloride ions across the membrane, Equation (4-4) must be expanded to include the chloride current, i_{Cl}:

$$i_K + i_{Na} + i_{Cl} = 0 \qquad (4\text{-}5)$$

Equation (4-5) is, in fact, the starting point in the derivation of the Goldman equation (see Appendix B). Note that because of the negative charge of chloride and because of the electrical convention for the direction of current flow, an outward movement of chloride ions is actually an inward membrane current.

Factors Affecting Ionic Current Across a Cell Membrane

What factors govern the amount of current carried across the membrane by a particular ion? We would expect that one important factor would be the difference between the equilibrium potential for the ion and the actual membrane potential. As an example, consider the movement of potassium ions across the membrane. We know that if $E_m = E_K$, there is a balance between the electrical and concentrational forces for potassium and there is no net movement of potassium across the membrane. In this situation, then, $i_K = 0$. As shown in Figure 4-2, if E_m does not equal E_K, the resulting imbalance in electrical and concentrational forces will drive a net movement of potassium across the membrane. The larger the difference between E_m and E_K, the larger the imbalance between the electrical and concentration gradients and the larger the net movement of potassium. Thus, i_K depends on $E_m - E_K$. This difference is called the **driving force** for membrane current carried by an ion.

We would also expect that the permeability of the membrane to an ion would be an important determinant of the amount of membrane current carried by that ion. If the permeability is high, the ionic current at a particular value of driving force will be higher than if the permeability were low. Thus, because p_K is much greater than p_{Na}, the potassium current resulting from a 10 mV difference between E_m and E_K will be much larger than the sodium current resulting from a 10 mV difference between E_m and E_{Na}. This is, in electrical terms, the reason why the steady-state membrane potential of a cell lies close to E_K rather than E_{Na}: In order for Equation (4-4) to be obeyed, the driving force for sodium entry $(E_m - E_{Na})$ must be much greater than the driving force for potassium exit $(E_m - E_K)$.

Membrane Permeability Versus Membrane Conductance

To place the discussion in the preceding section on more quantitative ground, it is necessary to introduce a new concept that is closely related to membrane permeability: **membrane conductance.** The conductance of a membrane to an ion is an index of the ability of that ion to carry current across the membrane: The higher the conductance, the greater the ionic current for a given driving force. Conductance is analogous to the reciprocal of the resistance of an electrical circuit to current flow: The higher the resistance of a circuit, the lower the amount of current that flows in response to a particular voltage. This behavior of electrical circuits can be conveniently summarized by Ohm's law: $i = V/R$. Here, i is the current flowing through a resistor, R, in the presence of a voltage gradient, V. The equivalent form for the flow of an ionic current across a membrane is, using potassium as an example, as follows:

$$i_K = g_K(E_m - E_K) \tag{4-6}$$

where g_K is the conductance of the membrane to potassium ions. The unit of electrical conductance is siemens, abbreviated S; a 1 V battery will drive 1 ampere of current through a 1 S conductance. Similar equations can be written for sodium and chloride:

$$i_{Na} = g_{Na}(E_m - E_{Na}) \tag{4-7}$$

$$i_{Cl} = g_{Cl}(E_m - E_{Cl}) \tag{4-8}$$

Note that for the usual values of E_m (-71 mV), E_K (-80 mV), and E_{Na} ($+58$ mV), the potassium current is a positive number and the sodium current is a negative number, as required by the fact that the two currents flow in opposite directions across the membrane. By convention in neurophysiology, an outward membrane current (such as i_K, at the steady-state E_m) is positive and an inward current (such as i_{Na}, at the steady-state E_m) is negative.

The membrane conductance to an ion is closely related to the membrane permeability to that ion, but the two are not identical. The membrane current carried by a particular ion, and hence the membrane conductance to that ion, is proportional to the rate at which ions are crossing the membrane (that is, the ionic flux). That rate depends not only on the permeability of the membrane to the ion, but also on the number of available ions in the solution. As an example, imagine a cell membrane with many potassium channels (Figure 4-5). The permeability of this membrane to potassium is thus high. If there are few potassium ions in solu-

(A) High permeability + few ions = low ionic current

(B) High permeability + many ions = larger ionic current

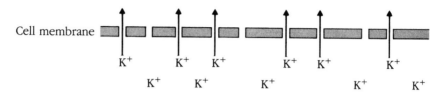

tion, however, the chance is small that a K^+ will encounter a channel and cross the membrane. In this case, the potassium current will be low and the conductance of the membrane to K^+ will be low even though the permeability is high. On the other hand, if there are many potassium ions available to cross the membrane (see Figure 4-5B), the chance that a K^+ will encounter a channel is high, and the rate of K^+ flow across the membrane will be high. The permeability remains fixed but the ionic conductance increases when more potassium ions are available. The point is that the potassium conductance of the membrane depends on the concentration of potassium at the membrane. For the most part, however, a change in permeability of a membrane to an ion produces a corresponding change in the conductance of the membrane to that ion. Thus, when we are dealing with changes in membrane conductance—as in the next chapter—we can treat a conductance change as a direct index of the underlying permeability change.

Figure 4-5
Illustration of the difference between permeability and conductance. (A) A cell membrane is highly permeable to potassium, but there is little potassium in solution. Therefore, the ionic current carried by potassium ions is small and the membrane conductance to potassium is small. (B) The same cell membrane in the presence of a higher potassium concentration has a larger potassium conductance because the potassium current is larger. The permeability, however, is the same as in (A).

Behavior of Single Ion Channels

At this point, it is worthwhile considering the properties of the ionic current flowing through an individual ion channel. We have already seen that the total membrane permeability of a cell to a particular ion depends on the number of channels the cell has that allow the ion to cross. But in addition, the total permeability also depends on how readily ions go through a single channel.

In Equations (4-6) through (4-8), we showed that the ionic current across a membrane is equal to the product of the electrical driving force and the membrane conductance. Similar considerations apply to the ionic current flowing through a single open ion channel, and we can write (for a potassium channel, for example) the following:

$$i_S = g_S(E_m - E_K) \tag{4-9}$$

where i_S is the single-channel current and g_S is the single-channel conductance for the potassium channel in question. Analogous equations could be written for single sodium or chloride channels.

What would we expect to see if we could measure directly the electrical current flowing through a single ion channel in a cell membrane? Up to now, we have treated ion channels as simple open pores or holes that allow ions to cross the membrane. But real ion channels show somewhat more complex behavior: The protein molecule that makes up the channel can apparently exist in two conformational states, one in which the pore is open and ions are free to move through it, and one in which the pore is closed and ions are not allowed through. (Actually, channels frequently show more than two functional states, but for our purposes in this book, we can treat channels as being either open or closed.) Thus, channels behave as though access to the pore is controlled by a "gate" that can be open or closed; for this reason, we refer to the opening and closing of the channel as **channel gating**. The electrical behavior of such a gated ion channel is illustrated in Figure 4-6, which shows the electrical current we would measure through a small patch of cell membrane containing a single potassium channel. We find that when the channel is in the closed state, there is no current across the membrane patch because potassium ions have no path across the membrane; however, when the channel protein abruptly undergoes a transition to the open state, an outward current will suddenly appear as potassium ions begin to exit the cell through the open pore. When the channel makes a transition back to the closed state, the current will abruptly disappear again. As we will see in the next section of this book, the control of ion channel gating, and thus of the ionic conductance of the cell membrane, is an important way in which biological signals are passed both within a cell and between cells.

The amplitude of the current that flows through the open chan-

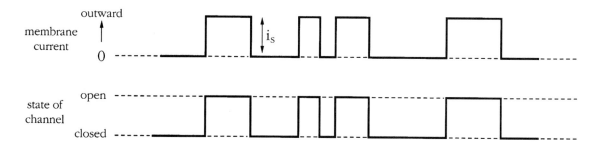

nel will be given by Equation (4-9); that is, the single-channel current will depend on the electrical driving force and on the single-channel conductance. How big is the single-channel current in real life? That depends on exactly what particular kind of ion channel we are talking about, because there is considerable variation in single-channel conductance among the various kinds of channels we encounter in a cell membrane (however, all of the individual channels of a particular kind would have the same single-channel conductance). But a value of about 20 pS might be considered typical (pS is the abbreviation for picosiemens, or 10^{-12} siemens). If the conductance is 20 pS and the driving force is 50 mV, then Equation (4-9) tells us that the single-channel current would be 10^{-12} A (or 1 pA; this corresponds to about 6 million monovalent ions per second). A small current indeed! Nevertheless, it has proved possible, using a measurement technique called the patch clamp, to measure directly the electrical current flowing through a single open ion channel. This technique, invented by Erwin Neher and Bert Sakmann, is discussed in more detail in Chapter 7. The ability to make such measurements from single channels has revolutionized the study of ion channels and made possible a great deal of what we know about how channels work.

What is the relationship between the total conductance of the cell membrane to an ion [Equations (4-6) to (4-8)] and the single-channel conductance? If, for example, a cell has only one type of potassium channel with single-channel conductance g_S, then the total membrane conductance to potassium, g_K, would be given by the following:

$$g_K = Ng_SP_o \qquad (4\text{-}10)$$

where N is the number of potassium channels in the entire cell membrane and P_o is the average proportion of time that an indi-

Figure 4-6
The electrical current flowing through a single potassium channel. The bottom trace shows the state of the channel (either open or closed), and the top trace shows the resulting ionic current through the channel. At the beginning of the trace, the channel is closed and so there is no ionic current flowing. When the channel opens, potassium ions begin to exit the cell through the channel, carrying an outward membrane current. The magnitude of the current (i_S) is given by Equation (4-9).

vidual channel is in the open state. You can see that if the individual channels are always closed, then P_o is zero and g_K would also be zero. Conversely, if individual channels are always open, then P_o is 1 and g_K will simply be the sum of all the individual single-channel conductances (i.e., $N \times g_S$).

Summary

In real cells, the resting membrane potential is the point at which sodium influx is exactly balanced by potassium efflux. This point depends on the relative membrane permeabilities to sodium and potassium; in most cells p_K is much higher than p_{Na} and the balance is struck close to E_K. The Goldman equation gives the quantitative expression of the relation between membrane potential on the one hand and ion concentrations and permeabilities on the other. Because the steady-state membrane potential lies between the equilibrium potentials for sodium and potassium, there is a constant exchange of intracellular potassium for sodium. This would lead to a progressive decline of the ionic gradients across the membrane if it were not for the action of the sodium-potassium pump. Thus, metabolic energy, in the form of ATP used by the pump, is required for the long-term maintenance of the sodium and potassium gradients. In the absence of chloride pumping, the chloride equilibrium potential will change to come into line with the value of membrane potential established by sodium and potassium. In some cells, however, a chloride pump maintains the internal chloride concentration in a nonequilibrium state, just as the sodium-potassium pump maintains internal sodium and potassium concentrations at nonequilibrium values.

The steady fluxes of potassium and sodium ions constitute electrical currents across the cell membrane, and at the steady-state E_m these currents cancel each other so that the net membrane current is zero. The membrane current carried by a particular ion is given by an ionic form of Ohm's law—that is, by the product of the driving force for that ion and the membrane conductance to that ion. The driving force is the difference between the actual value of membrane potential and the equilibrium potential for that ion. Conductance is a measure of the ability of the ion to carry electrical current across the membrane, and it is closely related to the membrane permeability to the ion.

Individual ion channels behave as though access to the pore through which ions can cross the membrane is controlled by a gate that may be open or closed. When the gate is open, the channel conducts and electrical current flows across the membrane; when the gate is closed, there is no current flow. The current through a single open channel is again given by the ionic form of Ohm's law—that is, the driving force multiplied by the single-channel conductance.

CELLULAR PHYSIOLOGY OF NERVE CELLS

Part I of this book focused on general properties that are shared by all cells. Every cell must achieve osmotic balance, and all cells have an electrical membrane potential. Part II considers properties that are peculiar to particular kinds of cells: those capable of modulating their membrane potential in response to stimulation from their environment. These cells are called **excitable** cells because they can generate active electrical responses that can serve as signals or triggers for other events. The most notable examples of excitable cells are the cells of the nervous system, which are called neurons.

The nervous system must receive information from the external environment and from the internal environment (that is, from the body), transmit and analyze that information, and coordinate an appropriate action in response. These functions of the nervous system range from controlling digestion in the gut of a worm to the complex processing your brain is performing in reading these words. As far as we know, however, the underlying signals the nervous system uses to process information are the same in the worm and in the human brain. In all cases, the signals passed along in the nervous system are electrical signals, modulations of the membrane potential.

Part II pertains to these electrical signals, the currency of information in the nervous system. We discuss how the signals arise, how a signal can be made to propagate throughout a nerve cell, and how the signals are passed along from one nerve cell to another. We will find that simple modifications of the scheme for the origin of the membrane potential presented in Chapter 4 can explain how neurons are capable of carrying out the vital signaling functions that are the task of the nervous system.

Generation of Nerve Action Potential

To set the stage for the discussion of the generation and transmission of signals in the nervous system, it is useful to review the characteristics of those signals within a well-defined example: the **patellar reflex**. This is better known as the knee-jerk reflex and is familiar to most of us. It is a type of stretch reflex and is elicited by a sudden stretching of the quadriceps muscle at the front of the thigh. The neural circuitry that underlies the patellar reflex is diagrammed in Figure 5-1. A sharp blow to the patellar tendon, which connects the knee cap (patella) to the bones of the lower leg, pulls the knee cap down and stretches the quadriceps muscle. Special sensory neurons with endings in the muscle are activated by the stretch. The message that the muscle has been stretched travels from the muscle along the thin fibers of the sensory neurons, which terminate in the lower spinal cord. Activity in the sensory neurons is then passed along to other neurons in the spinal cord. Among these neurons are motor neurons, each of which sends a long, thin fiber back to the thigh to make contact with the quadriceps muscle. Activity in the motor neurons causes the muscle to contract.

Neurons are structurally complex cells, with long fibrous extensions that are specialized to receive and transmit information throughout the nervous system. This complexity can be appreciated by looking at the delicate structure of a motor neuron, shown schematically in Figure 5-2A. The cell body, or **soma**, of the motor neuron—where the nucleus resides—is only a small part of the cell. It is typically only about 20 to 30 μm in diameter in the motor neurons involved in the patellar reflex. The soma gives rise, however, to a tangle of profusely branching processes

61

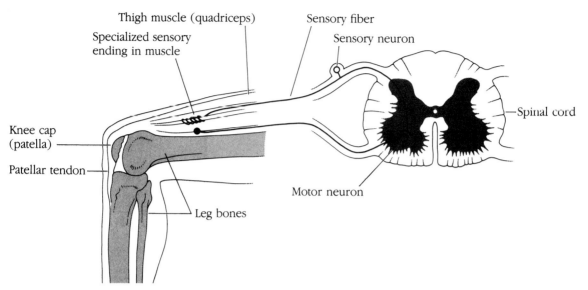

Thigh muscle (quadriceps)

Specialized sensory
ending in muscle

Sensory fiber

Sensory neuron

Spinal cord

Knee cap
(patella)

Patellar tendon

Leg bones

Motor neuron

Figure 5-1
Schematic representation of the
patellar reflex. The sensory
neuron is activated by stretching
the thigh muscle and in turn
activates motor neurons in the
spinal cord. Activity in the motor
neuron causes contraction of the
thigh muscle.

called **dendrites**, which might spread out for several millimeters
within the spinal cord. The dendrites are specialized to receive
signals passed along as the result of the activity of other neurons,
such as the sensory neurons of the patellar reflex, and to funnel
those signals along to the soma. The soma also gives rise to a thin
fiber, the **axon**, that is specialized to transmit activity from the
neuron to other neurons, or in the case of the motor neuron, to
the cells of the muscles. In some neurons, the axon may also
branch profusely and carry signals to many parts of the nervous
system. As shown in Figure 5-2B, the sensory neuron of the patellar reflex is structurally much simpler than the motor neuron.
Its soma, which is located just outside the spinal cord in the **dor-
sal root ganglion**, gives rise to only a single process. This process bifurcates to form the axon that carries the signal generated
by stretch from the muscle into the spinal cord.

In this chapter, we are concerned only with the long-distance
signal, the action potential, that carries the message along the
axon of the sensory neuron from the muscle to the spinal cord
and along the axon of the motor neuron from the spinal cord to
the muscle. This chapter concentrates on a descriptive introduction to the action potential and its mechanism; Chapter 6 presents
in more advanced form the elegant physiological experiments that
gave rise to the current view of that mechanism. In later chapters,
we discuss how the activity is transmitted from the sensory neuron to the motor neuron and how the muscle contracts in response to the activity of the motor neuron.

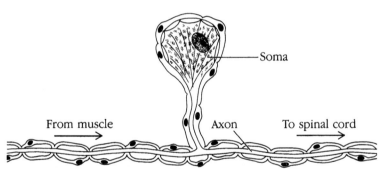

Figure 5-2
Structures of single neurons involved in the patellar reflex. (A) Motor neuron within spinal cord. (B) Sensory neuron just outside spinal cord.

The Action Potential

Ionic Permeability and Membrane Potential

In Chapter 4, we learned that membrane potential is governed by the relative permeabilities of the permeant ions. If the sodium permeability of a cell is greater than the potassium permeability, the membrane potential will be closer to E_{Na} than to E_K. Conversely, if a cell has greater potassium than sodium permeability, E_m will lie closer to E_K. In all cases discussed so far, ionic perme-

Figure 5-3

Example of an action potential in a neuron. (A) Experimental arrangement for recording the membrane potential of a nerve cell fiber. (B) Resting membrane potential and an action potential recorded via a voltage-sensing probe inside the sensory neuron of the patellar reflex loop. (C) Actual intracellular recordings from a single stretch-receptor sensory fiber during stretch of the muscle. The lower trace shows a single action potential on an expanded time scale, to show its waveform in more detail. (Traces in part C were redrawn from unpublished data kindly provided by R. Rose, M. Sedivec, and L. M. Mendell of the State University of New York at Stony Brook.)

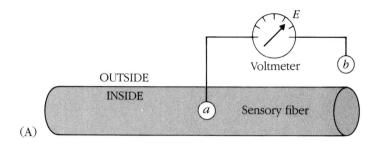

ability has been treated as a fixed characteristic of the cell membrane. In this chapter, however, we will see that the ionic permeability of the plasma membrane of excitable cells can vary. Specifically, we will see that a transient, dramatic increase in sodium permeability underlies the generation of the basic signal of the nervous system, the action potential.

Measuring the Long-Distance Signal in Neurons

What kind of signal carries the message along the sensory neuron in the patellar reflex? As mentioned earlier, the signals in the nervous system are electrical signals, and to monitor these signals it is necessary to measure the changes in electrical potential associated with the activation of the reflex. This can be done by placing an ultrafine probe inside the sensory axon and using this probe to measure the electrical membrane potential of the neuron. A diagram illustrating this kind of experiment is shown in Figure 5-3. A voltmeter has been connected to measure the voltage difference between point *a*, at the tip of the ultrafine probe, and point *b*, a reference point in the ECF. As shown in Figure 5-3B, when the probe is outside the sensory axon, both the probe and the reference point are in the ECF, and there is no voltage difference measured by the voltmeter. When the probe is inserted into the sensory fiber, however, we measure the voltage difference between the inside and outside of the neuron, the membrane potential. In neurophysiology, this process of measuring the transmembrane voltage of a cell is called intracellular recording, and the ultrafine probe is called an intracellular electrode. As expected from the discussion in Chapter 4, the membrane potential of the sensory fiber is about −70 mV.

When the muscle is stretched (see Figure 5-3B), something dramatic happens to the measured membrane potential in the sen-

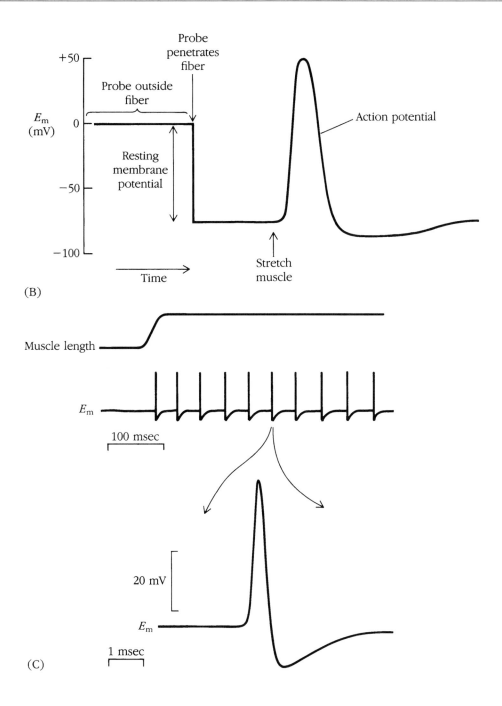

(B)

(C)

sory fiber. After a small delay, there is a sudden jump in membrane potential in which the potential transiently moves in a positive direction (a depolarization) and actually reverses in sign for a brief period, with the voltage settings inside the fiber becoming more positive than the outside. When the potential returns toward its resting value, it may transiently become more negative than its normal resting value. The transient jump in potential is called an action potential, which is the long-distance signal of the nervous system. If the stretch is sufficiently strong, it might elicit a series of several action potentials, each with the same shape and amplitude. Figure 5-3C shows actual examples of action potentials recorded via an intracellular electrode inside a sensory axon during stretch of a muscle.

Characteristics of the Action Potential

The action potential has several important characteristics that will be explained in terms of the underlying ionic permeability changes. These include the following:

1. Action potentials are triggered by depolarization. The stimulus that initiates an action potential in a neuron is a reduction in the membrane potential, that is, a depolarization of the membrane. Normally, the depolarization is produced by some external stimulus, such as the stretching of the muscle in the case of the sensory neuron in the patellar reflex, or by the action of another neuron, as in the transmission of excitation from the sensory neuron to the motor neuron in the patellar reflex.

2. A threshold level of depolarization must be reached in order to trigger an action potential. A small depolarization from the normal resting membrane potential will not produce an action potential. In most neurons, it is necessary to depolarize the membrane by about 10 to 20 mV in order to trigger an action potential; therefore, if a neuron has a resting membrane potential of about -70 mV, we would probably have to reduce the membrane potential to about -60 to -50 mV in order to trigger an action potential.

3. Action potentials are all-or-none events. This means that once a stimulus is strong enough to reach threshold, the amplitude of the action potential is independent of the strength of the stimulus. In other words, the amplitude and form of the action potential are fixed: The event either occurs all the way (if a depolarization is above threshold) or it doesn't occur at all (if the depolarization is below threshold). In this manner, the triggering of an action potential is like the firing of a gun: The speed with which the bullet leaves the barrel is independent of whether the trigger was pulled softly or hard.

4. *An action potential propagates without decrement throughout a neuron, but it does so at a speed much slower than the rate at which electricity propagates through a wire.* Figure 5-3 shows intracellular recordings of the action potentials triggered in a sensory neuron by stretching the quadriceps muscle. If we recorded simultaneously from the sensory fiber at two locations, one near the muscle and the other near the spinal cord, we would find that the action potential at the two locations has the same amplitude and form. Thus, as the signal travels from the muscle—where it originated—to the spinal cord, its amplitude remains unchanged. However, there would be a significant delay, almost 0.1 second, between the appearance of the action potential near the muscle and its arrival at the spinal cord. The conduction speed in a typical mammalian nerve fiber is about 10 to 20 m/sec, although speeds as high as 100 m/sec have been observed.

5. *At the peak of the action potential, the membrane potential reverses sign, becoming inside positive.* As shown in Figure 5-3, the membrane potential during an action potential transiently overshoots zero, so that the inside of the cell becomes positive with respect to the ECF for a brief time. This is called the overshoot of the action potential. When the action potential repolarizes toward the normal resting membrane potential, it transiently becomes more negative than normal. This is called the undershoot of the action potential.

6. *After a neuron fires an action potential, there is a brief period, called the absolute refractory period, during which it is impossible to make the neuron fire another action potential.* The absolute refractory period varies somewhat from one neuron to another, but it usually lasts about 1 msec. This sets a maximum limit of about 1000 action potentials per second on the rate at which a neuron can fire.

The goal of the remainder of this chapter is to explain all of these characteristics of the nerve action potential in terms of the underlying changes in the ionic permeability of the cell membrane and the resulting movements of ions.

Initiation and Propagation of Action Potentials

Some of the fundamental properties of action potentials can be studied experimentally using an apparatus like that diagrammed in Figure 5-4A. Imagine that a long section of a single axon is removed and arranged in the apparatus so that intracellular probes can be placed inside the fiber at two points, *a* and *b*, which are 10 cm apart. The probe at *a* is set up to pass positive or negative charge into the fiber and to record the resulting change in membrane potential, while the probe at *b* records membrane potential only. The effect of injecting negative charge at a constant rate at *a* is shown in Figure 5-4B. The extra negative charges make the interior of the fiber more negative, and the membrane potential increases; that is, the membrane is hyperpolarized. At the same time, the probe at *b* records no change in membrane potential at all. This is because the plasma membrane is leaky to charge: It is not a very good electrical insulator. In Chapter 3, we discussed the cell membrane as an electrical capacitor. In addition, the membrane behaves like an electrical resistor; that is, there is a direct path through which ionic current may flow across the membrane. As we saw in Chapter 4, that current path is through the ion channels inserted into the lipid bilayer of the plasma membrane. Thus, the charges injected at *a* do not travel very far down the fiber before leaking out of the cell across the plasma membrane. None of the charges reaches *b*, and so there is no change in membrane potential at *b*. When we stop injecting negative charges at *a*, all the injected charge leaks out of the cell, and the membrane potential returns to its normal resting value.

Another way of looking at the situation in Figure 5-4B is in terms of the flow of electrical current. The negative charges injected into the cell at a constant rate constitute an electrical current originating from the experimental apparatus. The return path

Figure 5-4
Demonstration of action potential generation and propagation in a segment of a nerve fiber. (A) Apparatus for recording electrical activity of a segment of a sensory nerve fiber. The probes at points *a* and *b* allow recording of membrane potential, and the probe at *a* also allows charges to be injected into the fiber. (B) Injecting negative charges at *a* causes a hyperpolarization at *a*. All injected charges leak out across the membrane before reaching *b*, and there is no change in membrane potential at *b*. (C) Injection of a small amount of positive charge produces a depolarization at *a* that again does not reach *b*. (D) If a stronger depolarization is induced at *a*, an action potential is generated. The action potential propagates without decrement along the fiber and is recorded at full amplitude at *b*.

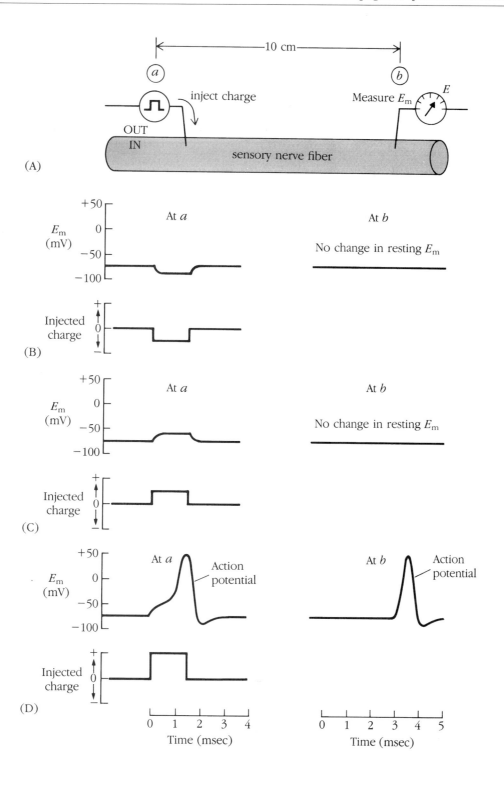

for the current to the apparatus lies in the ECF, so that in order to complete the circuit the current must exit across the plasma membrane. Two paths are available for the current at the point where it is injected: It can flow across the membrane immediately or it can move down the axon to flow out through a more distant segment of axon membrane. This situation is illustrated in Figure 5-5. The injected current will thus divide, some taking one path and some the other. The proportion of current taking each path depends on the relative resistances of the two paths: More current will flow down the path with less resistance. With each increment in distance along the axon, that fraction of the injected current that flowed down the axon again faces two paths: It can continue down the interior of the axon or it can cross the membrane at that point. The current will again divide, and some fraction of the fraction of the injected current will continue down the nerve fiber. This will continue until all the injected current has crossed the membrane, and no current is left to flow further down the interior of the axon. At that point, the injected current will not influence the membrane potential because there will be no remaining injected current. Thus, the change in membrane potential produced by current injection (see Figure 5-4A) decays with distance from the injection site. The greatest effect occurs at the injection site, and there is progressively less effect as injected current is progressively lost across the plasma membrane. The cell membrane is not a particularly good insulator (it has a low resistance to current flow compared, for example, with the insulator surrounding the electrical wires in your house), and the ICF inside the axon is not a particularly good conductor (its resistance to current flow is high compared with that of a copper wire). This set of circumstances favors the rapid decay of injected current with distance. In real axons, the hyperpolarization produced by current injected at a point decays by about 95% within 1 to 2 mm of the injection site.

Let's return now to the experiment shown in Figure 5-4. The effect of injecting positive charges into the axon is shown in Figure 5-4C. If the number of positive charges injected is small, the effect is simply the reverse of the effect of injecting negative charges; the membrane depolarizes while the charges are injected, but the effect does not reach *b*. When charge injection ceases, the extra positive charges leak out of the fiber, and membrane potential returns to normal. If the rate of injection of positive charge is increased, as in Figure 5-4D, the depolarization is larger. If the depolarization is sufficiently large, an all-or-none ac-

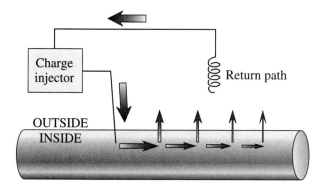

Figure 5-5
Schematic representation of the decay of injected current in an axon with distance from the site of current injection.

tion potential, like that recorded when the muscle was stretched (see Figure 5-3), is triggered at *a*. Now, the probe at *b* records a replica of the action potential at *a*, except that there is a time delay between the occurrence of the action potential at *a* and its arrival at *b*. Thus, action potentials are triggered by depolarization, not by hyperpolarization (characteristic 1, above); the depolarization must be large enough to exceed a threshold value (characteristic 2); and the action potential travels without decrement throughout the nerve fiber (characteristic 4). What ionic properties of the neuron membrane can explain these properties?

Changes in Relative Sodium Permeability During an Action Potential

The key to understanding the origin of the action potential lies in the discussion in Chapter 4 of the factors that influence the steady-state membrane potential of a cell. Recall that the resting E_m for a neuron will lie somewhere between E_K and E_{Na}. According to the Goldman equation, the exact point at which it lies will be determined by the ratio p_{Na}/p_K. As we saw in Chapter 4, p_{Na}/p_K of a resting neuron is about 0.02, and E_m is near E_K.

What would happen to E_m if sodium permeability suddenly increased dramatically? The effect of such an increase in p_{Na} is diagrammed in Figure 5-6. In the example, p_{Na} undergoes an abrupt thousandfold increase, so that $p_{Na}/p_K = 20$ instead of 0.02. According to the Goldman equation, E_m would then swing from about -70 mV to about $+50$ mV, near E_{Na}. When p_{Na}/p_K returns to 0.02, E_m will return to its usual value near E_K. Note that the swing in membrane potential in Figure 5-6 reproduces qualita-

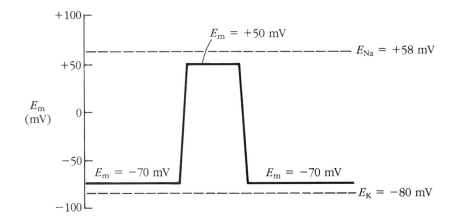

Figure 5-6
The relation between relative sodium permeability and membrane potential. When the ratio of sodium to potassium permeability (upper trace) is changed, the position of E_m relative to E_K and E_{Na} changes accordingly.

tively the change in potential during an action potential. Indeed, a transient increase in sodium permeability, as in Figure 5-6, is responsible for the swing in membrane polarization from near E_K to near E_{Na} and back during an action potential.

Voltage-Dependent Sodium Channels of the Neuron Membrane

Recall that ions must cross the membrane through transmembrane pores or channels. A dramatic increase in sodium permeability like that shown in Figure 5-6 requires a dramatic increase in the number of membrane channels that allow sodium ions to enter the cell. Thus, the resting p_{Na} of the membrane of an excitable cell is only a small fraction of what it could be because most membrane sodium channels are closed at rest. What stimulus causes these hidden channels to open and produces the positive swing of E_m during an action potential? It turns out that the conducting state of sodium channels of excitable cells depends on

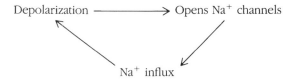

Figure 5-7
Explosive cycle leading to the depolarizing phase of an action potential.

the membrane potential. When E_m is at the usual resting level or more negative, these sodium channels are closed, Na^+ cannot flow through them, and p_{Na} is low. These channels open, however, when the membrane is depolarized. The stimulus for opening of the voltage-dependent sodium channels of excitable cells is a reduction of the membrane potential.

Because the voltage-dependent sodium channels respond to depolarization, the response of the membrane to depolarization is regenerative, or explosive. This is illustrated in Figure 5-7. When the membrane is depolarized, p_{Na} increases, allowing sodium ions to carry positive charge into the cell. This depolarizes the cell further, causing a greater increase in p_{Na} and more depolarization. Such a process is inherently explosive and tends to continue until all sodium channels are open and the membrane potential has been driven up to near E_{Na}. This explains the all-or-none behavior of the nerve action potential: Once triggered, the process tends to run to completion.

Why should there be a threshold level of depolarization? Under the scheme just discussed, it might seem that any small depolarization would set the action potential off. However, in considering the effect of a depolarization, we must take into account the total current that flows across the membrane in response to the depolarization, not just the current carried by sodium ions. Recall that at the resting E_m, p_K is very much greater than p_{Na}; therefore, flow of K^+ out of the cell can counteract the influx of Na^+ even if p_{Na} is moderately increased by a depolarization. Thus, for a moderate depolarization, the efflux of potassium might be larger than the influx of sodium, resulting in a net outward membrane current that keeps the membrane potential from depolarizing further and prevents the explosive cycle underlying the action potential. In order for the explosive process to be set in motion and an action potential to be generated, a depolarization must produce a net inward membrane current, which will in turn produce a further depolarization. A depolarization that produces an action potential must be sufficiently large to open quite a few sodium channels in order to overcome the efflux of potassium ions resulting from the depolarization. The **threshold potential** will be reached at that value of E_m where the influx of Na$^+$ exactly balances the efflux of K$^+$; any further depolarization will allow Na$^+$ influx to dominate, resulting in an explosive action potential.

Factors that influence the actual value of the threshold potential for a particular neuron include the density of voltage-sensitive sodium channels in the plasma membrane and the strength of the connection between depolarization and opening of those channels. Thus, if voltage-sensitive sodium channels are densely packed in the membrane, opening only a small fraction of them will produce a sizable inward sodium current, and we would expect that the threshold depolarization would be smaller than if the channels were sparse. Often, the density of voltage-sensitive sodium channels is highest just at the point (called the **initial segment**) where a neuron's axon leaves the cell body; this results in that portion of the cell having the lowest threshold for action potential generation. Another important factor in determining the threshold is the steepness of the relation between depolarization and sodium channel opening. In some cases the sodium channels have "hair triggers," and only a small depolarization from the resting E_m is required to open large numbers of channels. In such cases we would expect the threshold to be close to the resting membrane potential. In other neurons, larger depolarizations are necessary to open appreciable numbers of sodium channels, and the threshold is farther from resting E_m.

Repolarization

What causes E_m to return to rest again following the regenerative depolarization during an action potential? There are two important factors: (1) the depolarization-induced increase in p_{Na} is transient; and (2) there is a delayed, voltage-dependent increase in p_K. These are discussed in turn below.

The effect of depolarization on the voltage-dependent sodium channels is twofold. These effects are summarized by the diagram in Figure 5-8, which illustrates the behavior of a single voltage-sensitive sodium channel in response to a depolarization. The channel acts as though the flow of Na$^+$ is controlled by two independent gates. One gate, called the m gate, is closed when E_m is equal to or more negative than the usual resting potential. This gate thus prevents Na$^+$ from entering the channel at the resting potential. The other gate, called the h gate, is open at the usual

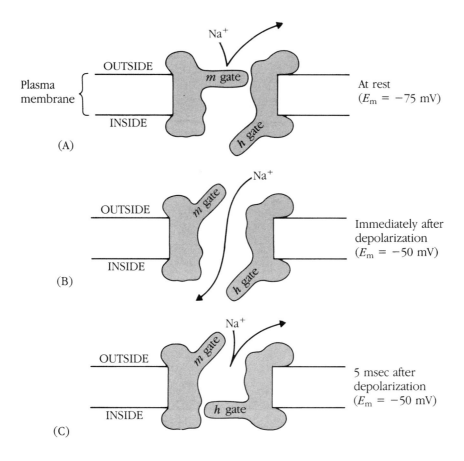

Plasma membrane

OUTSIDE

m gate

Na⁺

INSIDE

h gate

(A)

At rest
($E_m = -75$ mV)

OUTSIDE

m gate

Na⁺

INSIDE

h gate

(B)

Immediately after depolarization
($E_m = -50$ mV)

OUTSIDE

m gate

Na⁺

INSIDE

h gate

(C)

5 msec after depolarization
($E_m = -50$ mV)

Figure 5-8
Schematic representation of the behavior of a single voltage-sensitive sodium channel in the plasma membrane of a neuron. (A) The state of the channel at normal resting membrane potential. (B) Upon depolarization, the *m* gate opens rapidly and sodium ions are free to move through the channel. (C) After a brief delay, the *h* gate closes, returning the channel to a nonconducting state.

resting E_m. Both gates respond to depolarization, but with different speeds and in opposite directions. The *m* gate opens rapidly in response to depolarization; the *h* gate closes in response to depolarization, but does so slowly. Thus, immediately after a depolarization, the *m* gate is open, allowing Na⁺ to enter the cell, but the *h* gate has not had time to respond to the depolarization and is thus still open. A little while later (about a millisecond or two), the *m* gate is still open, but the *h* gate has responded by closing, and the channel is again closed. The result of this behavior is that p_{Na} first increases in response to a depolarization, then declines again even when the depolarization is maintained in some way. This delayed decline in sodium permeability upon depolarization is called **sodium channel inactivation**. As shown in Figure 5-6, this return of p_{Na} to its resting level would alone be sufficient to bring E_m back to rest.

In addition to the voltage-sensitive sodium channels, there are

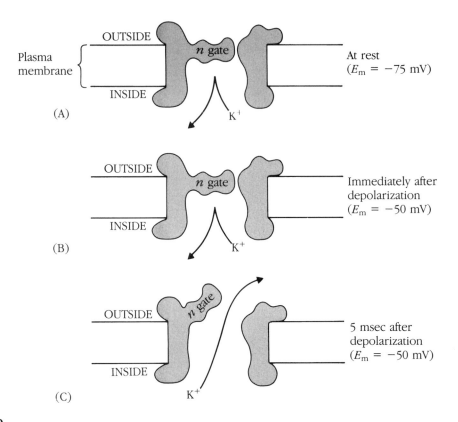

Figure 5-9

The behavior of a single voltage-sensitive potassium channel in the plasma membrane of a neuron. (A) At the normal resting membrane potential, the channel is closed. (B) Immediately after a depolarization, the channel remains closed. (C) With a delay, the *n* gate opens, allowing potassium ions to cross the membrane through the channel. The channel remains open as long as depolarization is maintained.

voltage-sensitive potassium channels in the membranes of excitable cells. These channels are also closed at the normal resting membrane potential. Like the sodium channel *m* gates, the gates on the potassium channels open upon depolarization, so that the channel begins to conduct K^+ when the membrane potential is reduced. However, the gates of these potassium channels, which are called *n* gates, respond slowly to depolarization, so that p_K increases with a delay following a depolarization. The characteristic behavior of a single voltage-sensitive potassium channel is shown in Figure 5-9. Unlike the sodium channel, there is no gate on the potassium channel that closes upon depolarization; the channel remains open as long as the depolarization is maintained and closes only when membrane potential returns to its normal resting value.

These voltage-sensitive potassium channels respond to the depolarizing phase of the action potential and open at about the time sodium permeability returns to its normal low value as *h* gates close. Therefore, the repolarizing phase of the action potential is produced by the simultaneous decline of p_{Na} to its resting level and increase of p_K to a higher than normal level. Note that during this time, p_{Na}/p_K is actually smaller than its usual resting value. This explains the undershoot of membrane potential below its resting value at the end of an action potential: E_m approaches closer to E_K because p_K is still higher than usual while p_{Na} has returned to its resting state. Membrane potential returns to rest as the slow n gates have time to respond to the repolarization by closing and returning p_K to its normal value.

The sequence of changes during an action potential is summarized in Figure 5-10, and characteristics of the various gates are summarized in Table 5-1. An action potential would be generated in the sensory neuron of the patellar reflex in the following way. Stretch of the muscle induces depolarization of the specialized sensory endings of the sensory neuron (probably by increasing the relative sodium permeability). This depolarization causes the m gates of voltage-sensitive sodium channels in the neuron membrane to open, setting in motion a regenerative increase in p_{Na}, which drives E_m up near E_{Na}. With a delay, h gates respond to the depolarization by closing and the n gates of the potassium channels respond by opening. The combination of these delayed gating events drives E_m back down near E_K and actually below the usual resting E_m. Again with a delay, the repolarization causes the h gates to open and the n gates to close, and the membrane returns to its resting state, ready to respond to any new depolarizing stimulus.

The scheme for the ionic changes underlying the nerve action potential was worked out in a series of elegant electrical experiments by A. L. Hodgkin and A. F. Huxley of Cambridge University. Chapter 6 describes those experiments and presents a quantitative version of the scheme shown in Figure 5-10.

The Refractory Period

The existence of a refractory period would be expected from the gating scheme summarized in Figure 5-10. When the h gates of the voltage-sensitive sodium channels are closed (states C and D in Figure 5-10), the channels cannot conduct Na^+ no matter what the state of the m gate might be. When the membrane is in this condition, no amount of depolarization can cause the cell to fire an action potential; the h gates would simply remain closed, preventing the influx of Na^+ necessary to trigger the regenerative explosion. Only when enough time has passed for a significant number of h gates to reopen will the neuron be capable of producing another action potential.

Table 5-1 Summary of responses of voltage-sensitive sodium and potassium channels to depolarization.

Type of channel	Gate	Response to depolarization	Speed of response
Sodium	*m* gate	Opens	Fast
Sodium	*h* gate	Closes	Slow
Potassium	*n* gate	Opens	Slow

Propagation of an Action Potential Along a Nerve Fiber

We can now see how an action potential arises as a result of a depolarizing stimulus, such as the muscle stretch in the case of the sensory neuron of Figure 5-1. How does that action potential travel from the ending in the muscle along the long, thin sensory fiber to the spinal cord? The answer to this question is inherent in the scheme for generation of the action potential just presented. As we've seen, the stimulus for an action potential is a depolarization of greater than about 10 to 20 mV from the normal resting level of membrane potential. The action potential itself is a depolarization much in excess of this threshold level. Thus, once an action potential occurs at one end of a neuron, the strong depolarization will bring the neighboring region of the cell above threshold, setting up a regenerative depolarization in that region. This will in turn bring the next region above threshold, and so on. The action potential can be thought of as a self-propagating wave of depolarization sweeping along the nerve fiber. When the sequence of permeability changes summarized in Figure 5-10 occurs in one region of a nerve membrane, it guarantees that the same gating events will be repeated in neighboring segments of

Figure 5-10
The state of voltage-sensitive sodium and potassium channels at various times during an action potential in a neuron. (A) At rest, neither channel is in a conducting state. (B) During the depolarizing phase of the action potential, sodium channels open, but potassium channels have not had time to respond to the depolarization. (C) During the repolarizing phase, sodium permeability begins to return to its resting level as *h* gates have sufficient time to respond to the depolarizing phase. At about the same time, potassium channels respond to the depolarization and open. (D) During the undershoot, sodium permeability has returned to its usual low level; potassium permeability, however, remains elevated because *n* gates respond slowly to the repolarization of the membrane. The resting state of the membrane is restored as *h* gates and *n* gates have time to respond to the repolarization.

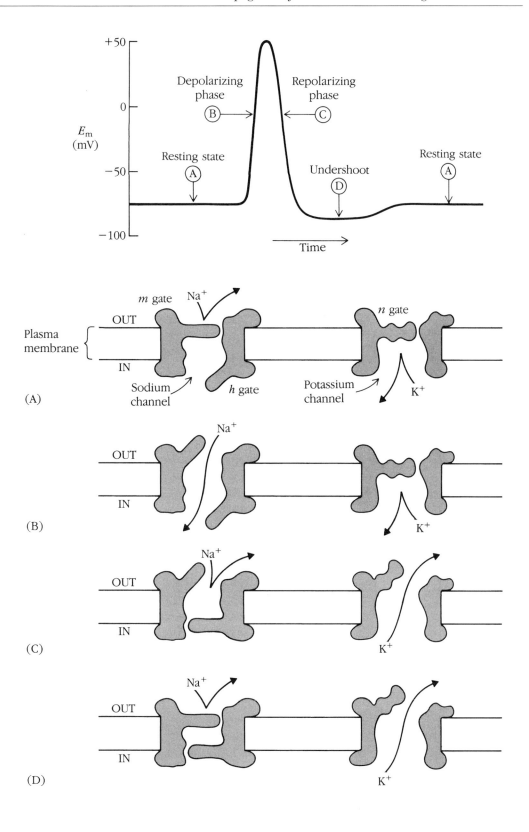

membrane. In this manner, the cyclical changes in membrane permeability, and the resulting action potential, chew their way along the nerve fiber from one end to the other, as each segment of axon membrane responds in turn to the depolarization of the preceding segment. This behavior is analogous to that of a lighted fuse, in which the heat generated in one segment of the fuse serves to ignite the neighboring segment.

A more formal description of propagation can be achieved by considering the electrical currents that flow along a nerve fiber during an action potential. Imagine that we freeze an action potential in time while it is traveling down an axon, as shown in Figure 5-11A. We have seen that at the peak of the action potential, there is an inward flow of current, carried by sodium ions. This is shown by the inward arrows at the point labeled 1 in Figure 5-11A. The region of axon occupied by the action potential will be depolarized with respect to more distant parts of the axon, like those labeled 2 and 3. This difference in electrical potential means that depolarizing current will be leaving the depolarized region and flowing along the inside of the nerve fiber; that is, positive charges will move out from the region of depolarization. In the discussion of the response to injected current in an axon (see Figures 5-4 and 5-5), we learned that a voltage change produced by injected current decayed with distance from the point of injection. Similarly, the depolarization produced by the influx of sodium ions during an action potential will decay with distance from the region of membrane undergoing the action potential. This decay of depolarization with distance reflects the progressive leakage of the depolarizing current across the membrane, which occurs because the membrane is a leaky insulator. Figure 5-11B illustrates the profile of membrane potential that might be observed along the length of the axon at the instant the action potential at point 1 reaches its peak. Note that there is a region of axon over which the depolarization, although decaying, is still above the threshold for generating an action potential in that part of the membrane. Thus, if we "unfreeze" time and allow events to move along, the region that is above threshold will generate its own action potential. This process will continue as the action potential sweeps along the axon, bringing each successive segment of axon above threshold as it goes.

The flow of depolarizing current from the region undergoing an action potential is symmetrical in both directions along the axon, as shown in Figure 5-11A. Thus, current flows from point

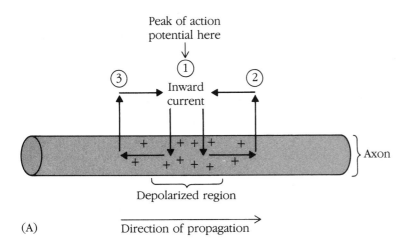

Peak of action
potential here

Inward
current

Axon

Depolarized region

(A)

Direction of propagation

Figure 5-11
The decay of depolarization with
distance from the peak of the
action potential at a particular
instant during the propagation of
the action potential from left to
right along the axon.

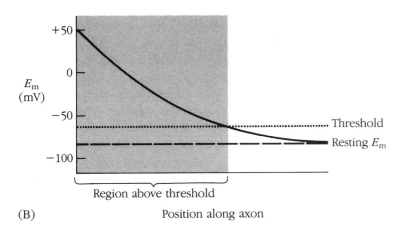

E_m
(mV)

+50

0

−50

−100

Threshold

Resting E_m

Region above threshold

(B)

Position along axon

1 to both point 2 and point 3 in the figure. Nevertheless, the action potential in an axon typically moves in only one direction. That is because the region the action potential has just traversed, like point 3, is in the refractory period phase of the action potential cycle and is thus incapable of responding to the depolarization originating from the action potential at point 1. Of course, if a neurophysiologist comes along with an artificial situation, like that shown in Figure 5-4, and stimulates an action potential in the middle of a nerve fiber, that action potential will propagate in both directions along the fiber. The normal direction of propagation in an axon—the direction taken by normally occurring action potentials—is called the **orthodromic** direction; an abnormal ac-

tion potential propagating in the opposite direction is called an **antidromic** action potential.

Factors Affecting the Speed of Action Potential Propagation

The speed with which an action potential moves down an axon varies considerably from one axon to another; the range is from about 0.1 m/sec to 100 m/sec. What characteristics of an axon are important in determining the velocity of the propagation of an action potential? Examine Figure 5-11B again. Clearly, if the rate at which the depolarization falls off with distance is less, the region of axon brought above threshold by an action potential at point 1 will be larger. If the region above threshold is larger, then an action potential at a particular location will set up a new action potential at a greater distance down the axon and the rate at which the action potential moves down the fiber will be greater. The rate of voltage decrease with distance will in turn depend on the relative resistance to current flow of the plasma membrane and the intracellular path down the axon. Recall from the discussion of the response of an axon to the injection of current (see Figure 5-5) that there are always two paths that current flowing down the inside of an axon at a particular point can take: It can continue down the interior of the fiber or cross the membrane at that point. We said that the portion of the current taking each path depends on the relative resistances of the two paths. If the resistance of the membrane could be made higher or if the resistance of the path down the inside of the axon could be made lower, the path down the axon would be favored and a larger portion of the current would continue along the inside. In this situation, the depolarization resulting from an action potential would decay less rapidly along the axon; therefore, the rate of propagation would increase.

Thus, two strategies can be employed to increase the speed of action potential propagation: Increase the electrical resistance of the plasma membrane to current flow, or decrease the resistance of the longitudinal path down the inside of the fiber. Both strategies have been adopted in nature. Among invertebrate animals, the strategy has been to decrease the longitudinal resistance of the axon interior. This can be accomplished by increasing the diameter of the axon. When a fiber is fatter, it offers a larger cross-sectional area to the internal flow of current; the effective resistance of this larger area is less because the current has many parallel paths to choose from if it is to continue down the interior of the axon. For the same reason, the electric power company uses large-diameter copper wire for the cables leaving a power-generating station; these cables must carry massive currents and thus must have low resistance to current flow to avoid burning up. Some invertebrate axons are the neuronal equivalent of these power cables: Axons up to 1 mm in diameter are found in some invertebrates. As expected, these giant axons are the fastest-conducting nerve fibers of the invertebrate world.

Among vertebrate animals, there is also a large variation in the size of axons, ranging from less than 1 μm in diameter to as big as 30 to 50 μm in diameter. Thus, even the largest axons in a human nerve do not begin to rival the size of the giant axons of invertebrates. Nevertheless, the fastest-conducting vertebrate axons are actually faster than the giant invertebrate axons. Vertebrate animals have adopted the strategy of increasing the membrane resistance to current as well as increasing the internal diameter. This has been accomplished by wrapping the axon with extra layers of insulating cell membrane: In order to reach the exterior, electrical current must flow not only through the resistance of the axon membrane, but also through the cascaded resistance of the tightly wrapped layers of extra membrane. Figure 5-12A shows a schematic cross-section of a vertebrate axon wrapped in this way. The cell that provides the spiral of insulating membrane surrounding the axon is a type of **glial cell**, a non-neuronal supporting cell of the nervous system that provides a sustaining mesh in which the neurons are embedded.

The insulating sheath around the axon is called **myelin**. By increasing the resistance of the path across the membrane, the myelin sheath forces a larger portion of the current flowing as the result of voltage change to move down the interior of the fiber. This increases the spatial spread of a depolarization along the axon and increases the rate at which an action potential propagates. In order to set up a new action potential at a distant point along the axon, however, the influx of sodium ions carrying the depolarizing current during the initiation of the action potential must have access to the axon membrane. To provide that access, there are periodic breaks in the myelin sheath, called **nodes of Ranvier**, at regular intervals along the length of the axon. This is diagrammed in Figure 5-12B. Thus, the depolarization resulting from an action potential at one node of Ranvier spreads along the interior of the fiber to the next node, where it sets up a new action

Figure 5-12
Propagation of an action
potential along a myelinated
nerve fiber. (A) Cross-section of
a myelinated axon, showing the
spiral wrapping of the glial cell
membrane around the axon.
(B) The depolarization from an
action potential at one node
spreads far along the interior of
the fiber because the insulating
myelin prevents the leakage of
current across the plasma
membrane.

Glial cell

Axon

(A)

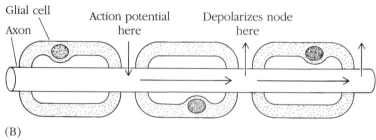

Glial cell

Axon

Action potential
here

Depolarizes node
here

(B)

potential. The action potential leaps along the axon, jumping from
one node to the next. This form of action potential conduction is
called **saltatory conduction**, and it produces a dramatic im-
provement in the speed with which a thin axon can conduct an
action potential along its length.

The myelin sheath also has an effect on the behavior of the
axon as an electrical capacitor. Recall from Chapter 3 that the cell
membrane can be viewed as an insulating barrier separating two
conducting compartments (the ICF and ECF). Thus, the cell membrane forms a capacitor. The capacitance, or charge-storing ability, of a capacitor is inversely related to the distance between the
conducting plates: The smaller the distance, the greater the number of charges that can be stored on the capacitor in the presence
of a particular voltage gradient. Thus, when the myelin sheath
wrapped around an axon increases the distance between the conducting ECF and ICF, the effective capacitance of the membrane
decreases. This means that a smaller number of charges needs to
be added to the inside of the membrane in order to reach a par-

ticular level of depolarization. (If it is unclear why this is true, review the calculation in Chapter 3 of the number of charges on a membrane at a particular voltage.) An electrical current is defined as the rate of charge movement—that is, the number of charges per second. In the presence of a particular depolarizing current, then, a given level of voltage will be reached faster on a small capacitor than on a large capacitor. Because the myelin makes the membrane capacitance smaller, a depolarization will spread faster, as well as farther, in the presence of myelin.

Molecular Properties of the Voltage-Sensitive Sodium Channel

Ion channels are proteins, and like all proteins, the sequence of amino acids making up the protein of a particular ion channel is coded by a particular gene. Thus, it is possible to study the properties of ion channels by applying techniques of molecular biology to isolate and analyze the corresponding gene. This has been done for an increasing variety of ion channels, including the voltage-sensitive sodium channel that underlies the action potential. The sodium channel is a large protein, containing some 2000 individual amino acids. A model of how the protein folds up into a three-dimensional structure has been developed, and this model is summarized schematically in Figure 5-13. According to the model, the protein consists of four distinct regions, called domains. Each domain consists of six separate segments that extend all the way across the plasma membrane (transmembrane segments), which are labeled S1 through S6. Within a domain, then, the protein threads its way through the membrane six times (see Figure 5-13). The amino acid sequences of each of the six transmembrane segments within a particular domain are similar to the corresponding segments in the other domains. Thus, the overall structure of the channel can be thought of as a series of six transmembrane segments, repeated four times.

It is thought that the four domains aggregate in a circular pattern, as shown in Figure 5-13B, to form the pore of the channel. The lining of the pore determines the permeation properties of the channel and gives the channel its selectivity for sodium ions. Interestingly, it seems that the lining is actually made up of the external loop connecting segments S5 and S6 within each of the four domains. In order for this external loop to form the transmembrane pore through which sodium ions cross the membrane,

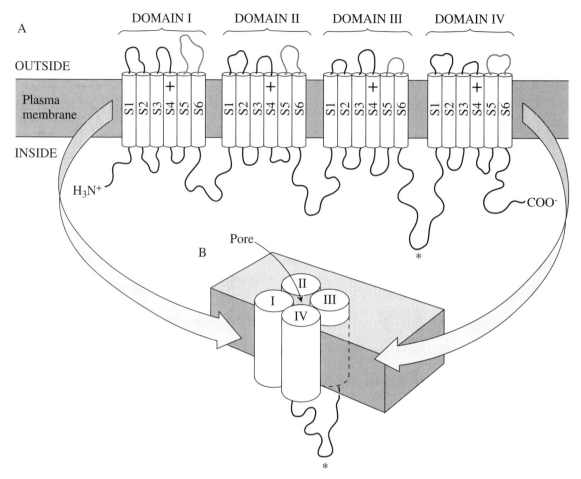

Figure 5-13
Molecular structure of the voltage-sensitive sodium channel. (A) The linear structure of the molecule. It consists of four domains of similar make-up, labeled with Roman numerals; each domain has six transmembrane segments (S1–S6). The highly positively charged segment S4 is indicated in each domain by a plus sign. The asterisk indicates the linkage between domains III and IV, which is involved in inactivation gating. In (A), the domains are shown in a linear arrangement, for clarity. In reality, the domains likely form a circular arrangement with the pore at the center, as shown in (B). The extracellular loop shown between S5 and S6 in (C) may fold in as indicated, to line the entry to the pore and thus control the ionic selectivity of the channel.

it must fold down into the pore in the manner shown schematically in Figure 5-13C.

One important question about the channel is what part of the protein is responsible for detecting changes in the membrane potential and thus imparts voltage sensitivity to the channel. Here, attention has focused on the fourth transmembrane segment of each domain, segment S4, which is marked with a plus sign in

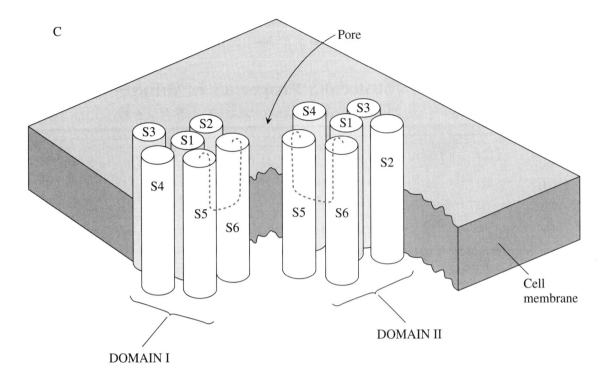

Figure 5-13A. Segment S4 has an unusual accumulation of positive charge (because of positively charged arginine and lysine residues in that part of the protein), which should give S4 high sensitivity to the electrical field across the membrane. Also, the positive charges in S4 are located within the membrane, which is the correct position to be acted upon by the transmembrane voltage. To test the idea that the charges in S4 are the voltage sensors, W. Stühmer and co-workers constructed artificial sodium channels by altering the DNA so that one or more of the arginines or lysines in S4 was replaced with a neutral or negatively charged amino acid. These artificial channels were less voltage dependent than the normal channels, suggesting that the charges in S4 are indeed the voltage sensors that detect depolarization of the membrane and activate the opening of the *m* gate.

Another important issue is to establish the identity of the sodium inactivation gate, the *h* gate. Here, Stühmer and co-workers found that the part of the protein connecting domains III and IV (marked with an asterisk in Figure 5-13) is important. When that region was deleted or altered, the inactivation process was greatly impaired, though activation seemed normal. Note that this part of the protein is on the intracellular side of the membrane, which is where we have drawn the *h* gate in our cartoon diagrams of sodium channels in earlier figures in this chapter.

Molecular Properties of Voltage-Dependent Potassium Channels

The DNA coding for various other voltage-activated channels, including voltage-activated potassium channels, has also been analyzed to reveal the sequence of amino acids making up those proteins. It is interesting that these voltage-activated channels have similar (though, of course, not identical) amino acid sequences, especially in segment S4, which seems to impart the voltage sensitivity. Thus, voltage-activated channels of various kinds represent a family of proteins coded by related genes that probably arose during the course of evolution from a single ancestral ion-channel gene that existed eons ago. Potassium channel genes, however, encode proteins that are much smaller than sodium channels. In fact, the protein encoded by potassium channel genes seems to correspond to a single one of the four domains present in the voltage-activated sodium channel (see Figure 5-13). It is thought that functional potassium channels are formed by the aggregation of four of these individual protein subunits, so that the whole channel has an arrangement similar to that of the sodium channel shown in Figure 5-13B. In the sodium channel, however, the four domains are combined together into one large, continuous protein molecule, whereas in potassium channels each domain consists of a separate protein subunit.

Calcium-Dependent Action Potentials

Action potentials are not unique to neurons. Action potentials are also found in non-neuronal excitable cells, such as muscle cells (as we will see in Part III of this book), and even in single-celled animals. Figure 5-14A shows that the paramecium, a protozoa, can produce action potentials similar to those of nerve cells, except that the action potential results from an influx of calcium ions rather than sodium ions as in the typical nerve action potential. The depolarizing upstroke of the action potential is caused by an influx of positively charged calcium ions, rather than an influx of sodium ions. As with sodium ions, the equilibrium potential for calcium ions (with a valence of +2) is positive, so if the membrane potential is negative and a calcium channel opens, there will be an influx of calcium into the cell. In the case of the sodium-dependent action potential, sodium channels activated by depolarization provide the basis for the regenerative all-or-none depolarizing phase of the action potential. Similarly, in the case of calcium-dependent action potentials, calcium channels that open upon depolarization underlie the depolarizing phase of the action potential. Depolarization opens calcium channels, which allow the influx of positively charged calcium ions, which in turn produces more depolarization and opens more calcium channels (see Figure 5-7 for the analogous situation with depolarization-activated sodium channels). The calcium-dependent action potential in paramecium is also similar to nerve action potentials in that it serves a coordinating function: It regulates the direction of ciliary beating and thus the movement of the cell. Mutant paramecia that lack the ion channels underlying the calcium action potential are unable to reverse the direction of ciliary beating and thus are unable to swim backward when they encounter noxious environmental stimuli. Because these mutants can only swim forward, they are called "pawn" mutants, after the chess piece that can only move forward. Thus, some of the basic molecular machinery for electrical signaling, one of the hallmarks of nervous system function, predates by far the origin of the first neuron. This suggests that neural signaling arose by the evolutionary modification of preexisting signaling mechanisms, found already in single-celled animals.

Voltage-dependent calcium channels are found in most neurons, and in some neurons, these voltage-activated calcium channels contribute significantly to the action potential. A comparison between the waveform of the sodium-dependent action potential and the waveform of an action potential with a component caused by calcium influx is shown in Figure 5-14B. Often, the depolarization produced by calcium influx is slower and more sustained than the more spike-like action potential due to sodium and potassium channels alone. This is because the voltage-activated calcium channels commonly inactivate more slowly than do voltage-activated sodium channels, so they produce a more sustained influx of positive charge, and thus a more prolonged depolarization. In neurons with a calcium-dependent component, then, the action potential has a rapid upstroke caused by the opening of sodium channels, followed by a longer-duration plateau phase caused by the voltage-dependent calcium channels.

The influx of calcium ions through voltage-dependent calcium channels has functional consequences beyond contributing to the

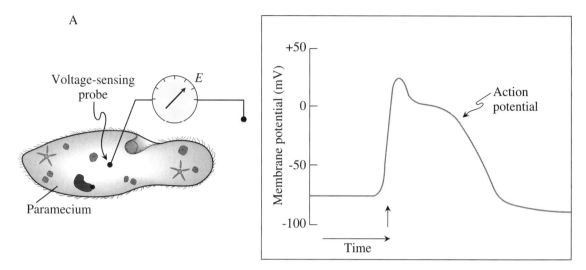

Figure 5-14

Calcium-dependent action potentials. (A) The single-celled protozoa, the paramecium, can produce an action potential similar to a nerve action potential. The diagram on the left shows the recording configuration for intracellular recording. The action potential elicited by an electrical stimulus (at the arrow) is shown on the right. (B) Comparison between action potentials in neurons without a contribution from voltage-dependent calcium channels (top) and those with a calcium component (bottom). The rising phase of the action potential on the bottom (black portion) is due to depolarization-activated sodium channels, and the dashed black line shows the expected time course of the action potential in the absence of calcium channels. The gray line shows the plateau depolarization caused by the opening of voltage-sensitive calcium channels.

action potential. The increase in the intracellular concentration of calcium that results from the influx is an important cellular signal that allows depolarization of a cell to be coupled to the triggering of internal cellular events. For example, we will see in Chapter 7 that an increase in intracellular calcium is the trigger for the release of neurotransmitter from the presynaptic terminal when an action potential arrives at the synaptic junction between two neurons. Another important effect of internal calcium is the activation of other kinds of ion channels. In addition to the potassium channels opened by depolarization, which we discussed previously in this chapter, neurons frequently have potassium channels that are opened by an increase in internal calcium. Such calcium-activated potassium channels can contribute to action potential repolarization in neurons that have a calcium component in the action potential (for example, see Figure 5-14B). As we discussed earlier, an increase in potassium permeability accounts in part for the repolarizing phase of the action potential and produces the hyperpolarizing undershoot after repolarization. This increase in potassium permeability can be accomplished with voltage-activated potassium channels or with calcium-activated potassium channels. The activation scheme for calcium-activated potassium channels is summarized in Figure 5-15.

One important functional difference between voltage activated and calcium-activated potassium channels is the amount of time the channels can remain open after the membrane potential has returned to its negative level at the end of the action potential. The action potential undershoot corresponds to the time after an

B

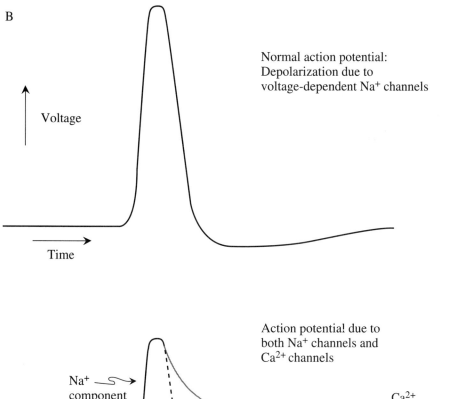

Voltage

Time

Normal action potential:
Depolarization due to
voltage-dependent Na+ channels

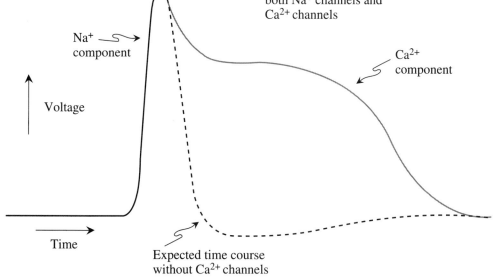

Na+
component

Voltage

Time

Action potential due to
both Na+ channels and
Ca²⁺ channels

Ca²⁺
component

Expected time course
without Ca²⁺ channels

action potential when the voltage-dependent potassium channels
remain open, while sodium permeability has returned to rest; because the ratio p_{Na}/p_K is therefore *smaller* than the usual value, the
membrane potential is driven even nearer to the potassium equilibrium potential than the normal resting potential. The period of

A

OUT
Cell membrane
IN

Ca²⁺

Voltage-activated
Ca²⁺ channel
(opened by depolarization)

Calcium-activated
K⁺ channels
(opened by internal Ca²⁺)

Ca²⁺

Ca²⁺

K⁺

B

Depolarization ⟶ Ca²⁺ channels open ⟶ Ca²⁺ influx

↓

Repolarization ⟵ K⁺ efflux ⟵ Ca²⁺-activated K⁺ channels open

Figure 5-15

Activation of potassium channels by internal calcium ions. (A) Upon depolarization, voltage-dependent calcium channels open and calcium ions enter the cell from the ECF. The calcium ions then bind to and open calcium-activated potassium channels, which allow potassium ions to exit from the cell. (B) Summary of the sequence of events leading to the activation of calcium-activated potassium channels.

hyperpolarization during the undershoot ends as the voltage-dependent potassium channels close in response to repolarization, which takes a few milliseconds or less. Calcium-activated potassium channels, however, remain open for as long as the intracellular calcium level remains elevated after the action potential. This can be hundreds of times longer than the undershoot produced by the voltage-dependent potassium channels, as shown in Figure 5-16. The longer-lasting hyperpolarization is called the **afterhyperpolarization** to distinguish it from the undershoot. The presence of an afterhyperpolarization requires both a significant calcium influx during the action potential (to produce an increase in internal calcium concentration) and significant numbers of calcium-activated potassium channels (to produce an increase in potassium permeability in response to the increase in internal calcium). Not all neurons possess these requirements and thus not all neurons show prolonged afterhyperpolarizations. In neurons that have only a small component of calcium influx during a single action potential, afterhyperpolarizations can still be observed if the cell fires a rapid burst of action potentials, because the internal cal-

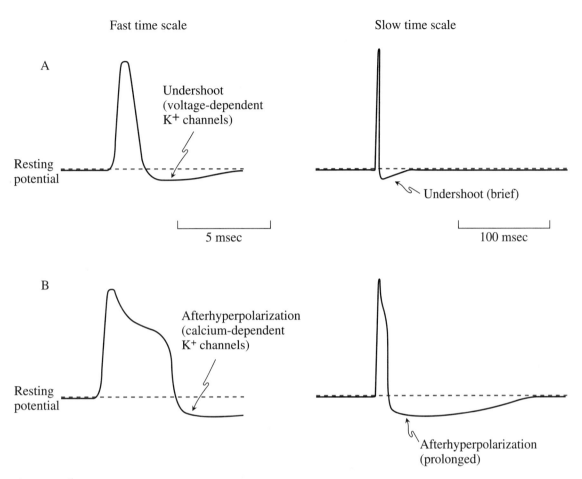

Figure 5-16
Time course of undershoot compared with the time course of afterhyperpolarization due to calcium-activated potassium channels. (A) Action potential of a neuron with only voltage-dependent sodium and potassium channels. (B) Action potential of a neuron with voltage-dependent calcium channels and calcium-activated potassium channels in addition to the usual voltage-dependent sodium and potassium channels. The traces on the left in both (A) and (B) show the action potential on a fast time scale (milliseconds), while the traces on the right show the same action potentials on a slower time scale (hundreds of milliseconds).

cium contributed by each action potential may sum temporally to reach the calcium level necessary to activate calcium-activated potassium channels. The afterhyperpolarization is important in determining the temporal patterning of action potentials, because the long period of increased potassium permeability makes it more difficult for the neuron to fire action potentials in a rapid series. In neurons that require a burst of several action potentials to initiate the afterhyperpolarization, the calcium-activated potassium channels can be important in terminating the burst. This can be a mechanism for timed bursts of action potentials separated by silent periods in neurons that control rhythmic events.

Summary

The basic long-distance signal of the nervous system is a self-propagating depolarization called the action potential. The action potential arises because of a sequence of voltage-dependent changes in the ionic permeability of the neuron membrane. This voltage-dependent behavior of the membrane is due to gated sodium and potassium channels. The conducting state of the sodium channels is controlled by m gates, which are closed at the usual resting E_m and open rapidly upon depolarization, and by h gates, which are open at the usual resting E_m and close slowly upon depolarization. The voltage-sensitive potassium channels are controlled by a single type of gate, called the n gate, which is closed at the resting E_m and opens slowly upon depolarization. In response to depolarization, p_{Na} increases dramatically as m gates open, and E_m is driven up near E_{Na}. With a delay, h gates close, restoring p_{Na} to a low level, and n gates open, increasing p_K. As a result, p_{Na}/p_K falls below its normal resting value, and E_m is driven back to near E_K. The resulting repolarization restores the membrane to its resting state.

The behavior of the voltage-dependent sodium and potassium channels can explain (1) why depolarization is the stimulus for the generation of an action potential, (2) why action potentials are all-or-none events, (3) how action potentials propagate along nerve fibers, (4) why the membrane potential becomes positive at the peak of the action potential, (5) why the membrane potential is transiently more negative than usual at the end of an action potential, and (6) the existence of a refractory period after a neuron fires an action potential.

Action potentials of some neurons have components contributed by voltage-dependent calcium channels, which open upon depolarization like voltage-dependent sodium channels but specifically allow an influx of calcium ions. The influx of calcium ions through these channels can increase the intracellular concentration of calcium. Calcium-activated potassium channels open when internal calcium is elevated, contributing to the repolarization of the action potential and producing a prolonged period of elevated potassium permeability during which the membrane potential is more negative than the usual resting membrane potential.

The Action Potential: Voltage-Clamp Experiments

In Chapter 5, we discussed the basic membrane mechanisms underlying the generation of the action potential in a neuron. We learned that all the properties of the action potential could be explained by the actions of voltage-sensitive sodium and potassium channels in the plasma membrane, both of which behave as though there are voltage-activated gates that control the permeation of ions through the channel. In this chapter, we discuss the experimental evidence that gave rise to this scheme for explaining the action potential. The fundamental experiments were performed by Alan L. Hodgkin and Andrew F. Huxley in the period from 1949 to 1952, with the participation of Bernard Katz in some of the early work. The Hodgkin-Huxley model of the nerve action potential is based on electrical measurements of the flow of ions across the membrane of an axon, using a technique known as voltage clamp. We start by describing how the voltage clamp works, and then we discuss the observations Hodgkin and Huxley made and how they arrived at the gated ion channel model discussed in the last chapter.

The Voltage Clamp

We saw in Chapter 5 that the permeability of an excitable cell membrane to sodium and potassium depends on the voltage across the membrane. We also learned that the voltage-induced permeability changes occur at different speeds for the different ionic "gates" on the voltage-sensitive channels. This means that the membrane permeability to sodium, for example, is a function of two variables: voltage and time. Thus, in order to study the permeability in a quantitative way, it is necessary to gain experimental control of one of these two variables. We can then hold that one variable constant and see how permeability varies as a function of the other variable. The voltage clamp is a recording technique that allows us to accomplish this goal. It holds membrane voltage at a constant value; that is, the membrane potential is "clamped" at a particular level. We can then measure the membrane current flowing at that constant membrane voltage and use the time course of changes in membrane current as an index of the time course of the underlying changes in membrane ionic conductance.

A diagram of the apparatus used to "voltage clamp" an axon is shown in Figure 6-1. Two long, thin wires are threaded longitudinally down the interior of an isolated segment of axon. One wire is used to measure the membrane potential, just as we did in a number of previous examples using intracellular microelectrodes; this wire is connected to one of the inputs of the voltage-clamp amplifier. The other wire is used to pass current into the axon and is connected to the output of the voltage-clamp amplifier. The other input of the amplifier is connected to an external voltage source, the command voltage, that is under the experimenter's control. The command voltage is so named because its value determines the value of the resting membrane potential that will be maintained by the voltage-clamp amplifier.

The amplifier in the voltage-clamp circuit is wired in such a way that it feeds a current into the axon that is proportional to the difference between the command voltage and the measured membrane potential, $E_C - E_m$. If that difference is zero (that is, if $E_m = E_C$), the amplifier puts out no current, and E_m will remain stable. If E_m does not equal E_C, the amplifier will pass a current into the axon to make the membrane potential move toward the command voltage. For example, if E_m is -70 mV and E_C is -60 mV, then $E_C - E_m$ is a positive number. Because the amplifier passes a current that is proportional to that difference, the current will also be positive. That is, the injected current will move positive charges into the axon and depolarize the membrane toward E_C. This would continue until the membrane potential equals the command potential of -60 mV. On the other hand, if E_C were more negative than E_m, $E_C - E_m$ would produce a negative number, and the injected current would be negative. In this case, the current would hyperpolarize the axon until the membrane potential equaled the command voltage.

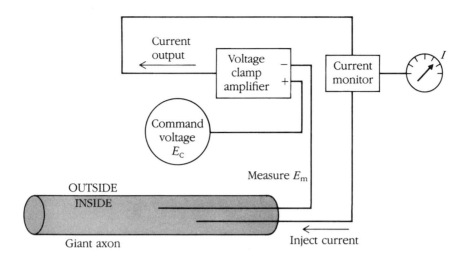

OUTSIDE

INSIDE

Giant axon

Measure E_m

Inject current

Figure 6-1
Schematic diagram of a voltage-clamp apparatus.

Measuring Changes in Membrane Ionic Conductance Using the Voltage Clamp

By inserting a current monitor into the output line of the amplifier, we can measure the amount of current that the amplifier is passing to keep the membrane voltage equal to the command voltage. How does this measured current give information about changes in ionic current and, therefore, changes in ionic conductance of the membrane? First of all, let's review what happens to membrane current and membrane potential without the voltage clamp, using the principles we discussed in Chapters 4 and 5. This is illustrated in Figure 6-2A, which shows the changes in transmembrane ionic current and membrane potential in response to a stepwise increase in p_{Na}, with p_K remaining constant. Under resting conditions, we have seen that the steady-state membrane potential will be between E_{Na} and E_K, at the membrane voltage at which the inward sodium current exactly balances the outward potassium current, so that the total membrane current is zero ($i_{Na} + i_K = 0$). When p_{Na} is suddenly increased, the steady state is perturbed, and there will be an increase in i_{Na}. This greater sodium influx causes E_m to move in a positive direction from its original resting value. With depolarization, however, potassium current increases because of the increasing difference between E_m and E_K. The membrane potential will reach a new steady state, governed by the new ratio of p_{Na}/p_K, at which both i_{Na} and i_K are larger than they were initially, but once again exactly balance each other. This is just a restatement of the basis of resting membrane potential discussed in detail in Chap-

A

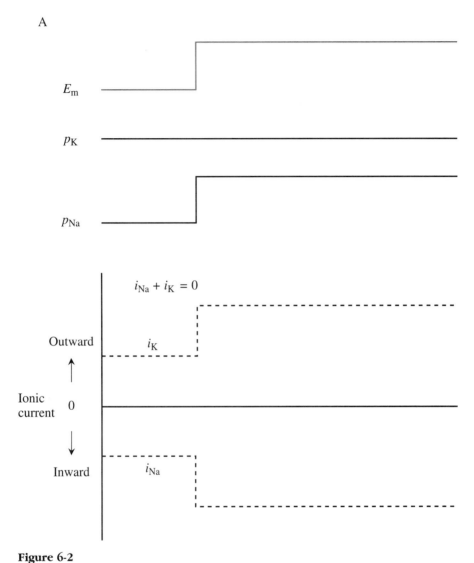

Figure 6-2
Ionic currents flowing in response to a stepwise change in p_{Na}, either without voltage clamp (A) or with voltage clamp (B). Without voltage clamp, both i_{Na} and i_K increase in response to the increase in p_{Na}, and a new steady-state membrane potential (gray trace) is reached at a more depolarized level. With voltage clamp, the membrane potential remains constant because the voltage-clamp apparatus injects current (i_{clamp}) that compensates for the increased sodium current. Potassium current remains constant because neither p_K nor E_m changes.

B

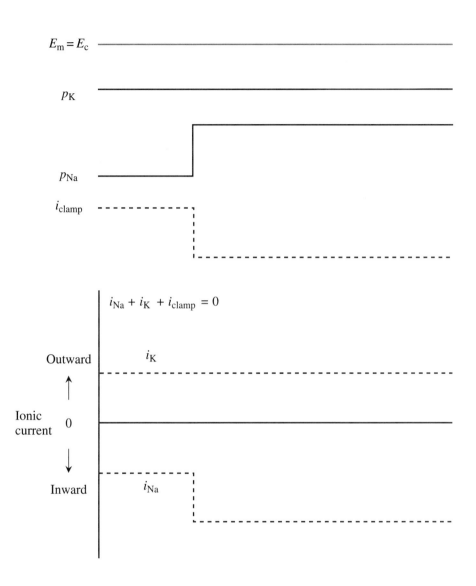

$i_{Na} + i_K + i_{clamp} = 0$

ter 4. Let's consider now what happens if the same change in p_{Na} occurs under voltage-clamp conditions, as shown in Figure 6-2B. Now we must consider an additional source of current: the current provided by the voltage-clamp apparatus (i_{clamp}). Suppose we set the command voltage, E_C, to equal the normal steady-state membrane potential of the cell and turn on the voltage-clamp apparatus. In this situation, E_m is already equal to E_C and the current injected by the voltage-clamp apparatus will be zero. Suppose that at some time after we turn on the apparatus, there is a sudden increase in the sodium permeability of the membrane. As we have just seen, this would normally cause the membrane potential to take up a new steady-state value closer to the sodium equilibrium potential; that is, the cell would depolarize because of the increase in inward sodium current across the membrane. However, now the voltage-clamp circuit will detect the depolarization as soon as it begins, and the voltage-clamp amplifier will inject negative current into the axon to counter the increased sodium current (see the trace labeled i_{clamp} in Figure 6-2B). The voltage clamp will continue to inject this holding current to maintain E_m at its usual resting value for as long as the increased sodium permeability persists, so that E_m remains equal to E_C. Thus, the injected current will be equal in magnitude to the increase in sodium current resulting from the increase in sodium permeability. Notice that there is now no change in i_K, because there is now no change in E_m (as well as no change in p_K). If the potassium permeability, rather than the sodium permeability, were to undergo a stepwise increase from its normal resting value, then the voltage-clamp apparatus will respond as shown in Figure 6-3. In this case, the increased potassium permeability would normally drive E_m more *negative*, toward E_K, and the cell would *hyperpolarize*. However, the voltage-clamp amplifier will inject a depolarizing current of the right magnitude to counteract the hyperpolarizing potassium current leaving the cell. The point is that the current injected by the voltage clamp gives a direct measure of the change in ionic current resulting from a change in membrane permeability to an ion.

How do we relate the measured change in membrane current to the underlying change in membrane permeability? Recall from Chapter 4 that the ionic current carried by a particular ion is given by the product of the membrane conductance to that ion and the voltage driving force for that ion, which is the difference between the actual value of membrane potential and the equilibrium potential for the ion. For example, for sodium ions

$$i_{Na} = g_{Na}(E_m - E_{Na}) \qquad (6\text{-}1)$$

Thus, we can calculate g_{Na} from the measured i_{Na} according to the relation

$$g_{Na} = i_{Na}/(E_m - E_{Na}) \qquad (6\text{-}2)$$

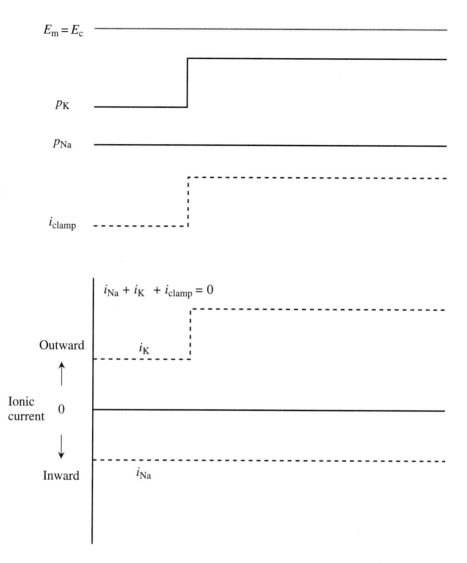

Figure 6-3
Changes in ionic current and injected current after a stepwise change in p_K under voltage clamp. Potassium current increases because of the increase in p_K, but the voltage-clamp amplifier injects compensating current to keep E_m constant.

In this calculation, E_m is equal to the value set by the voltage clamp, and E_{Na} can be computed from the Nernst equation or measured experimentally by setting E_C to different values and determining the setting that produces no change in ionic current upon a change in g_{Na} (that is, $E_m - E_{Na} = 0$). In this way, it is straightforward to obtain a measure of the time course of a change in membrane ionic conductance from the time course of the change in ionic current. As discussed in Chapter 4, conductance is not the same as permeability. However, for rapid changes in permeability like those underlying the action potential, we can treat the two as having the same time course.

The Squid Giant Axon

The experimental arrangement diagrammed in Figure 6-1 was technically feasible only because nature provided neurophysiology with an axon large enough to allow experimenters to thread a pair of wires down the inside. The axon used by Hodgkin and Huxley was the giant axon from the nerve cord of the squid. This axon can be up to 1 mm in diameter, large enough to be dissected free from the surrounding nerve fibers and subjected to the voltage-clamp procedure just described. The axon is so large that it is possible to squeeze the normal ICF out of the fiber—like toothpaste out of a tube—and replace it with artificial ICF of the experimenter's concoction. This allows the tremendous experimental advantage of being able to control the compositions of both the intracellular and the extracellular fluids.

Ionic Currents Across an Axon Membrane Under Voltage Clamp

The membrane currents flowing in a squid giant axon during a maintained depolarization can be studied in an experiment like that shown in Figure 6-4. In this experiment, the command voltage to the voltage-clamp amplifier is first set to be equal to the normal resting potential of the axon, which is about -60 to -70 mV. The command voltage is then suddenly stepped to -20 mV, driving the membrane potential rapidly up to the same depolarized value. A depolarization of this magnitude is well above threshold for eliciting an action potential in the axon; however, the voltage-clamp circuit prevents the membrane potential from undergoing the usual sequence of changes that occur during an action potential. The membrane potential remains clamped at -20 mV.

What current must the voltage-clamp amplifier inject into the axon in order to keep E_m at -20 mV? The sodium permeability of the membrane will increase in response to the depolarization and an increased sodium current will enter the axon through the increased membrane conductance to sodium. In the absence of the voltage clamp, this would set up a regenerative depolarization that would drive E_m up near E_{Na}, to about $+50$ mV. In order to counter this further depolarization, the voltage-clamp amplifier must inject a hyperpolarizing current during the strong depolarizing phase of the action potential. With time, however, the sodium permeability

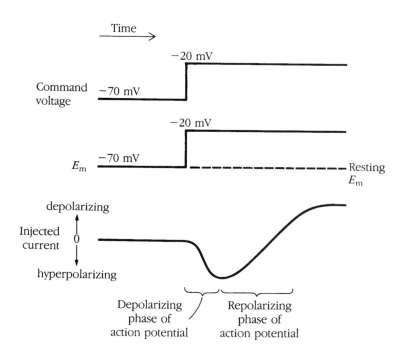

Figure 6-4
Diagram of the current injected by a voltage-clamp amplifier into an axon in response to a voltage step from −70 to −20 mV.

of the membrane declines, and the potassium permeability increases in response to the depolarization of the membrane. Normally, this would drive E_m back down near E_K. To counter this tendency and maintain E_m at −20 mV, the voltage clamp then must pass a depolarizing current that is maintained as long as potassium permeability remains elevated. Thus, in response to a depolarizing step above threshold, the membrane of an excitable cell would be expected to show a transient inward current followed by a maintained outward current. The voltage-clamp records of membrane current illustrating this sequence of changes are shown in Figure 6-4.

What was the nature of the evidence that the initial inward current was carried by sodium ions? This was demonstrated by measuring the membrane current resulting from a series of voltage steps of different amplitudes. As we demonstrated previously, if the clamped value of membrane potential were equal to the sodium equilibrium potential, there would be no driving force for a net sodium current across the membrane. Therefore, if the initial current is carried by sodium ions, that component of the current should disappear when the command voltage is equal to E_{Na}. A sample of membrane current observed in response to a voltage step to E_{Na} is shown in Figure 6-5. The initial component of in-

Figure 6-5

Diagram of the current injected by a voltage-clamp amplifier into an axon in response to a voltage step from the normal resting membrane potential to the sodium equilibrium potential. The initial sodium current is absent because there is no driving force for sodium current when E_m equals E_{Na}.

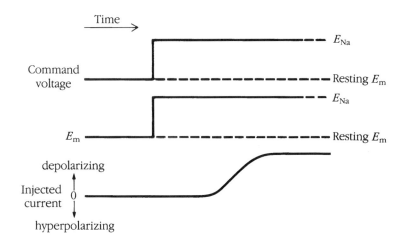

ward current disappears in this situation, leaving only the late outward current. Hodgkin and Huxley went one step further and systematically varied E_{Na} by altering the external sodium concentration; they found that the membrane potential at which the early current component disappeared was always E_{Na}. This is strong evidence that the inward component of current in response to a depolarization is carried by sodium ions. This notion also agrees with early observations that the membrane potential reached by the peak of the action potential was strongly influenced by the external sodium concentration.

The two components of membrane current can be separated by comparing the current observed following a voltage step to a particular voltage when that voltage is equal to E_{Na} and when E_{Na} has been moved to another value by altering the external sodium concentration. A specific example is shown in Figure 6-6. In this case, voltage-clamp steps are made to 0 mV in ECF containing normal sodium and in ECF with the sodium concentration reduced to be equal with the internal sodium concentration. In the normal-sodium ECF, E_{Na} will be positive to the command voltage; in the reduced-sodium ECF, E_{Na} will equal the command potential and there will be no net sodium current across the membrane. When the observed current in reduced-sodium ECF is subtracted from the current in normal-sodium ECF, the difference will be the sodium component of membrane current in response to a step depolarization to 0 mV. This isolated sodium current is shown in Figure 6-6C. The membrane currents in Figure 6-6C can be converted to membrane conductance according to Equation (6-2), and the result gives the time course of the membrane sodium and potas-

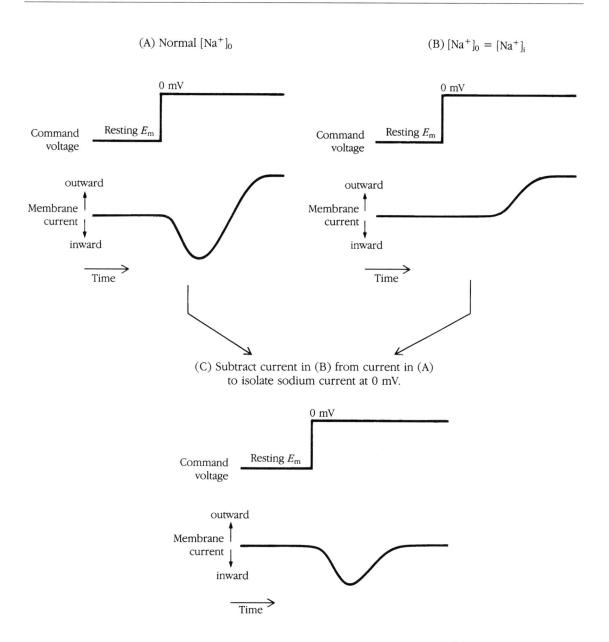

(A) Normal $[Na^+]_o$

(B) $[Na^+]_o = [Na^+]_i$

(C) Subtract current in (B) from current in (A)
to isolate sodium current at 0 mV.

Figure 6-6
Procedure for isolating the sodium component of the membrane current by varying the external sodium concentration to alter the sodium equilibrium potential.

sium conductances in response to a voltage-clamp step to 0 mV. This procedure can be repeated for a series of different values of command potential and E_{Na}, generating a full characterization of the sodium and potassium conductance changes as a function of both time and membrane voltage. The increase in sodium conductance in response to depolarization is transient, even if the depolarization is maintained. The increasing phase is called **sodium**

activation, and the delayed fall is called **sodium inactivation**. We discuss activation first and return later to the mechanism of inactivation. The onset of the increase in potassium conductance is slower than sodium activation and does not inactivate with maintained depolarization. Thus, at least on the brief time scale relevant to the action potential, potassium conductance remains high for the duration of the depolarizing voltage step.

This rather involved procedure has been simplified considerably by the discovery of specific drugs that block the voltage-sensitive sodium channels and other drugs that block the voltage-sensitive potassium channels. The sodium channel blockers most commonly used are the biological toxins tetrodotoxin and saxitoxin. Both seem to interact with specific sites within the aqueous pore of the channel and physically plug the channel to prevent sodium movement. Potassium channel blockers include tetraethylammonium (TEA) and 4-aminopyridine (4-AP). Thus, the isolated behavior of the sodium current could be studied by treating an axon with TEA, while the isolated potassium current could be studied in the presence of tetrodotoxin.

The Gated Ion Channel Model

Membrane Potential and Peak Ionic Conductance

Hodgkin and Huxley discovered that the peak magnitude of the conductance change produced by a depolarizing voltage-clamp step depended on the size of the step. This established the voltage dependence of the sodium and potassium conductances of the axon membrane. The form of this dependence is shown in Figure 6-7 for both sodium and potassium conductances. Note the steepness of the curves in both graphs. For example, a voltage step to -50 mV barely increases g_{Na}, but a step to -30 mV produces a large increase in g_{Na}. Hodgkin and Huxley suggested a simple model that could account for the voltage sensitivity of the sodium and potassium conductances. Their model assumes that many individual ion channels, each with a small ionic conductance, determine the behavior of the whole membrane as measured with the voltage-clamp procedure, and that each channel has two conducting states: an open state in which ions are free to cross through the pore, and a closed state in which the pore is blocked. That is, the channels behave as though access to the pore were controlled by a gate. The effect of membrane poten-

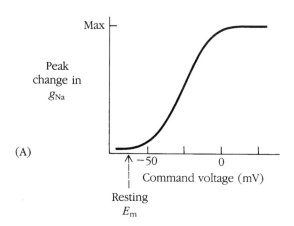

(A)

(B)

Figure 6-7
Voltage dependence of peak
sodium (A) and potassium (B)
conductances as a function of
the amplitude of a maintained
voltage step.

tial changes in this scheme is to alter the probability that a channel will be in the open, conducting state. With depolarization, the
probability that a channel is open increases, so that a larger fraction of the total population of channels is open, and the total
membrane conductance to that ion increases. The maximum conductance is reached when all the channels are open, so that further depolarization can have no greater effect.

In order for the conducting state of the channel to depend on
transmembrane voltage, some charged entity that is either part of
the channel protein or associated with it must control the access of
ions to the channel. When the membrane potential is near the resting value, these charged particles are in one state that favors closed
channels; when the membrane is depolarized, these charged particles take up a new state that favors opening of the channel. One
scheme like this is shown in Figure 6-8. The charged particles are

Figure 6-8

A schematic representation of the voltage-sensitive gating of a membrane ion channel. The conducting state of the channel is assumed in this model to depend on the binding of a charged particle to a site on the outer face of the membrane.

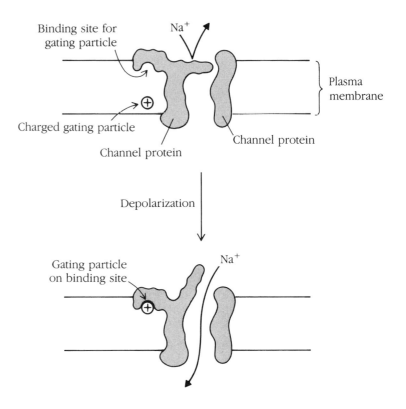

assumed to have a positive charge in Figure 6-8; thus, in the presence of a large, inside-negative electrical field across the membrane, most of the particles would likely be near the inner face of the membrane. Upon depolarization, however, the distribution of charged particles within the membrane would become more even, and the fraction of particles on the outside would increase. The channel protein in Figure 6-8 is assumed to have a binding site on the outer edge of the membrane that controls the conformation of the "gating" portion of the channel. When the binding site is unoccupied, the channel is closed; when the site binds one of the positively charged particles (called **gating particles**), the channel opens. Thus, upon depolarization, the fraction of channels with a gating particle on the binding site will increase, as will the total ionic conductance of the membrane. It is important to emphasize that the drawings in Figure 6-8 are illustrative only; it is not clear, for example, that the gating particles are positively charged, although evidence from molecular studies suggests so. Negatively charged particles moving in the opposite direction or a dipole rotating in the membrane could accomplish the same voltage-dependent gating function. The molecular mechanism underlying the change in conducting state of the channel protein is unknown at present. It seems likely, however, that a conformation change related to charge distribution within the membrane is involved.

The S-shaped relationship between ionic conductance and membrane potential shown in Figure 6-7 is as expected from basic physical principles for the movement of charged particles under the influence of an electrical field, as diagrammed schematically in Figure 6-8. The distribution of charged particles within the membrane will be related to the transmembrane electrical field (that is, the membrane potential) according to Boltzmann's relation:

$$P_o = \frac{1}{1 + e^{\left(\frac{W - z\epsilon E_m}{kT}\right)}} \tag{6-3}$$

where P_o is the proportion of positive gating particles on the outside of the membrane, z is the valence of the gating charge, ϵ is the electronic charge, E_m is membrane potential, k is the Boltzmann constant, T is the absolute temperature, and W is a voltage-independent term giving the offset of the relation along the voltage axis. The steepness of the rise in P_o with depolarization depends on the valence z of the gating charge: The larger z becomes, the steeper is the rise of P_o (and thus of conductance) with depolarization. As we noted earlier, the sodium and potassium conductances are steeply dependent on membrane potential, implying that the gating charge that moves in order to open a channel has a large valence. For example, to produce a rise in sodium conductance like that observed experimentally, the effective valence of the gating particle must be ~6 [that is, $z \approx 6$ in the Boltzmann relation of Equation (6-3)].

Kinetics of the Change in Ionic Conductance Following a Step Depolarization

We learned in Chapter 5 that differences in the speed with which the three types of voltage-sensitive gates respond to voltage changes are important in determining the form of the action potential. For instance, the opening of the potassium channels must be delayed with respect to the opening of the sodium channels to avoid wasteful competition between sodium influx and potassium efflux during the depolarizing phase of the action potential. We now consider how the time course, or kinetics, of the conductance changes fits into the charged gating particle scheme just presented.

Hodgkin and Huxley assumed that the rate of change in the membrane conductance to an ion following a step depolarization was governed by the rate of redistribution of the gating particles within the membrane. That is, they assumed that the interaction between gating particle and binding site introduced negligible delay into the temporal behavior of the channel. As an example, we consider the kinetics of opening of the sodium channel following a step depolarization. In formal terms, the movement of gating particles within the membrane can be described by the following first-order kinetic model:

$$m \underset{b_m}{\overset{a_m}{\rightleftharpoons}} (1 - m) \tag{6-4}$$

Here, m is the proportion of particles on the outside of the membrane, where they can interact with the binding sites, and $1 - m$ is the proportion of particles on the inside of the membrane. The rate constant, a_m, represents the rate at which particles move from the inner to the outer face of the membrane, and b_m is the rate of reverse movement. Because of the charge on the particles, a step change in the membrane voltage will cause an instantaneous change in the rate constants a_m and b_m. For instance, a step depolarization would increase a_m and decrease b_m, leading to a net increase in m and therefore a decrease in $1 - m$.

The equation governing the rate at which the charges redistribute following a change in membrane potential is as follows:

$$dm/dt = a_m(1 - m) - b_m m \tag{6-5}$$

In Equation (6-5), dm/dt is the net rate of change of the proportion of particles on the outside face of the membrane. In words, $a_m(1 - m)$ is the rate at which particles are leaving the inside of the membrane, and $b_m m$ is the rate at which particles are leaving the outside surface; the difference between those two rates is the net rate of change in m. If the distribution of particles is stable—as it would be if E_m had been constant for a long time—the rate at which particles move from inside to outside would equal the rate of movement in the opposite direction, and dm/dt would be zero. If the system is suddenly perturbed by a depolarization, a_m and b_m would change and the balance on the right side of Equation (6-5) would be destroyed. If the depolarization is maintained, the rate at which the system will approach a new steady distribution of particles will be governed by Equation (6-5).

The solution of a first-order kinetic expression like Equation (6-5) is an exponential function; that is, following a step change in membrane voltage m will approach a new steady value exponentially. The exponential solution can be written as follows:

$$m(t) = m_\infty - (m_\infty - m_0)e^{-(a_m + b_m)t} \qquad (6\text{-}6)$$

This equation states that following a change in membrane potential, m will change exponentially from its initial value (m_0) to its final value (m_∞) at a rate governed by the rate constants (a_m and b_m) for movement of the gating particles at that new value of membrane potential. The behavior of m with time after a depolarization, as expected from Equation (6-6), is summarized in Figure 6-9. The number of binding sites occupied by gating particles would be expected to be proportional to m, the fraction of available particles on the outer face of the membrane. Thus, if the occupation of a single binding site causes the channel to open and if the coupling between binding of the gating particle and opening of the channel involves no significant delays, the number of open channels would be expected to follow the same exponential time course as m after a step depolarization.

Because the total membrane sodium conductance is determined by the number of open sodium channels, sodium conductance measured with a voltage clamp would be expected to be exponential as well, given the assumption of a single gating particle leading to opening of the channel. This prediction, along with the actually observed kinetic behavior of g_{Na}, is diagrammed in Figure 6-10. Unlike the predicted exponential behavior, the rise in g_{Na} actually exhibited a pronounced delay following the voltage step. The S-shaped increase in g_{Na} would be explained if more than one binding site must be occupied by gating particles before the channel will open. If the binding to each of several sites is independent, the probability that any one site is occupied will be proportional to m and will thus rise exponentially with time after a step voltage change, as discussed already. The probability that all of a number of sites will be occupied will be the product of the probabilities that each single site will bind a gating particle. That is, if there are two binding sites, the probability that both are occupied will be the product of the probability that site 1 binds a particle and the probability that site 2 binds a par-

Figure 6-9
Change in the distribution of sodium channel gating particles after a depolarization of the membrane. (A) Schematic diagram of the distribution of charged gating particles at the normal resting potential and at different times after depolarization of the membrane. (B) The effect of a step change in membrane potential (top trace) on the rate constants for movement of the gating particles (middle traces) and on the proportion of particles on the outer side of the membrane (bottom trace).

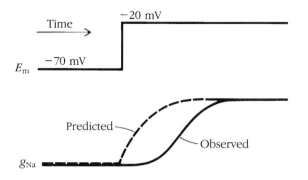

Figure 6-10
Predicted time course of the change in sodium conductance following a depolarizing step (dashed line), assuming that the proportion of open channels—and hence the total sodium conductance—is directly related to the fraction of gating particles on the outer face of the membrane. The solid line shows the observed change in sodium conductance following a step depolarization.

ticle. Because each of these probabilities is proportional to m, the joint probability that both sites are occupied is proportional to m^2. Similarly, if there were x sites, the probability of channel opening would be proportional to m^x. The actual rise in sodium conductance following a depolarizing step suggested that $x = 3$ for the sodium channel: Three binding sites must be occupied by gating particles before the channel will conduct. Thus, the turn-on of g_{Na} following a voltage-clamp step to a particular level of depolarization was proportional to m^3, and the temporal behavior of m was given by Equation (6-6).

A similar analysis was carried out for the change in potassium conductance following a step depolarization. The results suggested that $x = 4$ for the voltage-sensitive potassium channel of squid axon membrane. Thus, the gating charges for the potassium channel redistributed after a change in membrane potential according to a relation equivalent to Equation (6-5):

$$dn/dt = a_n(1 - n) - b_n n \qquad (6\text{-}7)$$

By analogy with the sodium system, n is the proportion of potassium gating particles on the outside of the membrane, $1 - n$ is the proportion on the inner face of the membrane, and a_n and b_n are the rate constants for particle transition from one face to the other. Equation (6-7) has a solution equivalent to Equation (6-6):

$$n(t) = n_\infty - (n_\infty - n_0)e^{-(a_n + b_n)t} \qquad (6\text{-}8)$$

Here, n_0 and n_∞ are the initial and final values of n. The rise in potassium conductance following a step depolarization was found to be proportional to n^4; therefore, the potassium channel behaves as though four binding sites must be occupied by gating particles in order for the gate to open. A major difference between the potassium and the sodium channels is that the rate constants a_n and b_n are smaller for potassium channels. That is, the sodium channel gating particles appear to be more mobile than their potassium channel counterparts; this accounts for the greater speed of the sodium channel in opening after a depolarization, which is a crucial part of the action potential mechanism.

Sodium Inactivation

Recall that the change in sodium conductance following a maintained depolarizing step is transient. We have so far considered only the first part of that change: the increase in sodium conductance called sodium activation. We now turn to the delayed decline in sodium conductance following depolarization. This delayed decline in conductance is called sodium inactivation. Following along in the manner used in the analysis of sodium and potassium channel opening, Hodgkin and Huxley assumed that sodium inactivation was caused by a voltage-sensitive gating mechanism. They supposed that the conducting state of the sodium channel was controlled by two gates: the activation gate whose opening we discussed already, and the inactivation gate. A diagram of this arrangement is shown in Figure 6-11. Like the activation gate, the inactivation gate is controlled by a charged gating particle; when the binding site on the gate is occupied, the inactivation gate is open. Unlike the activation gate, however, the inactivation gate is normally open and closes upon depolarization. If we keep the convention of the gating particle being positively charged, this behavior can be modeled by an arrangement with the inactivation gate and its binding site on the inner face of the membrane. Upon depolarization, the probability that a gating particle is on the inner face decreases, and so the probability that the gate closes will increase.

To study the voltage dependence of the sodium inactivation process, Hodgkin and Huxley performed the type of experiment illustrated in Figure 6-12. They used a fixed depolarizing test step of a particular amplitude and measured the peak amplitude of the increase in sodium conductance that resulted from the test step. The test depolarization was preceded by a long-duration prepulse whose amplitude could be varied. As shown in Figure 6-12, they found that a depolarizing prepulse reduced the amplitude of the response to the test depolarization, while a hyperpolarizing pre-

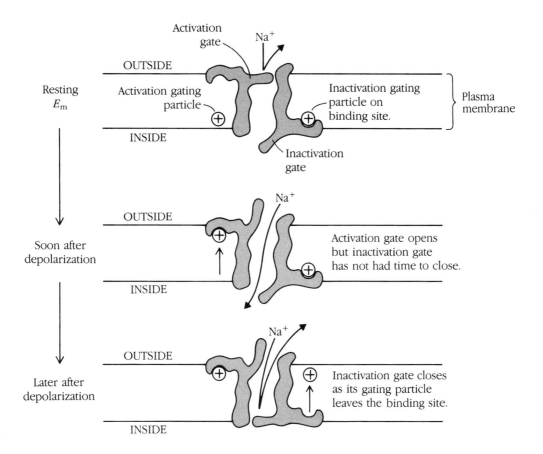

Figure 6-11
Diagram of the sodium channel
protein, showing effects of both
the activation and the
inactivation gates.

pulse increased the size of the test response. This implied that the depolarizing prepulses closed the inactivation gates of some portion of the sodium channels, so that those channels did not conduct even when the activation gates were opened by the subsequent depolarization; therefore, there was a smaller increase in sodium conductance during the test step. The finding that hyperpolarizing prepulses increased the test response suggests that the inactivation gates of some portion of the sodium channels are already closed at the normal resting potential; increasing E_m causes those gates to open, and the channels are then able to conduct in response to the test depolarization. By varying the amplitude of the prepulse, Hodgkin and Huxley were able to establish the dependence of the inactivation gate on membrane potential. The relation between E_m during the prepulse and the peak sodium conductance during the test depolarization is shown in Figure 6-13. Note that all the inactivation gates close when the membrane potential reaches about 0 mV, and that even a small depo-

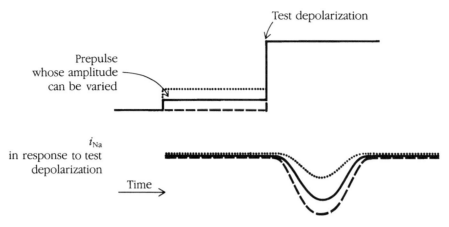

Figure 6-12

Procedure for measuring the voltage dependence of sodium inactivation.

Figure 6-13

Relation between the amplitude of an inactivating prepulse and the peak sodium conductance in response to a subsequent test depolarization.

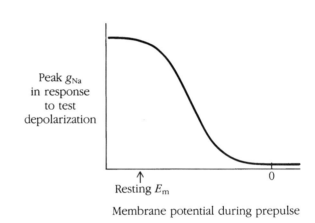

larization can cause a significant reduction in the peak change in sodium conductance.

The time course of sodium inactivation was studied by varying the duration of the prepulse, rather than its amplitude. With short prepulses, there was not much time for the inactivation gates to close, and the response to the test depolarization was only slightly reduced. With longer prepulses, there was a progressively larger effect. This relation between prepulse duration and peak sodium conductance during the test step is shown in Figure 6-14. It was found that the data were described by a single exponential equation, rather than the powers of exponentials that were necessary to describe the kinetics of sodium and potassium activation. Recall

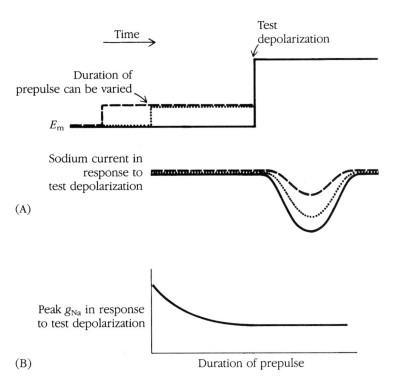

(A)

(B)

Figure 6-14
(A) Procedure for measuring the time course of sodium inactivation by varying the duration of depolarizing prepulses. (B) Resulting exponential time course of the closing of the inactivation gate of the sodium channel.

from the discussion of the voltage-dependent opening of the sodium channel that a single exponential is what would be expected if the state of the gate is controlled by a single gating particle. Thus, the closing of the inactivation gate seems to occur when a single particle comes off a single binding site on the gating mechanism. An equation analogous to Equations (6-6) and (6-8) can be written to describe the temporal behavior of the inactivation gate:

$$h(t) = h_\infty - (h_\infty - h_0)e^{-(a_h + b_h)t} \qquad (6\text{-}9)$$

In this case, however, the parameter h decreases with depolarization; that is, upon depolarization, h declines exponentially from its original value (h_0) to its final value (h_∞). The rate of that decline is governed by the rate constants, a_h and b_h, for movement of the inactivation gating particle through the membrane. As expected from the discussion in Chapter 5, the closing of the inactivation gate is slower than the opening of the activation gate, implying that the inactivation gating particle is less mobile (that is, the rate constants are smaller).

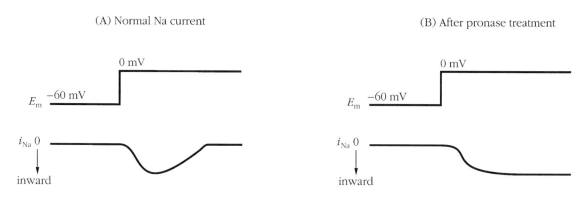

Figure 6-15

Removal of the inactivation gate by treating the inside of the membrane with a proteolytic enzyme, pronase. (A) Normal sodium current. The current rises (activates) and then declines (inactivates) during a maintained depolarization. (B) Sodium current after pronase treatment. The current activates normally, but fails to inactivate during a maintained depolarization.

Is there any reason to suppose that the activation and inactivation gates are separate entities, as drawn in Figure 6-11 and throughout Chapter 5? After all, we could get the same behavior of the channel with a single gate that first opens and then closes upon depolarization. There is evidence, however, that the processes of activation and inactivation of the sodium channel are controlled by distinct and separable parts of the channel protein molecule. If, for example, we apply a proteolytic enzyme, such as trypsin or pronase, to the intracellular membrane face, we can selectively eliminate sodium channel inactivation while leaving activation intact. The sodium current observed in such an experiment is shown in Figure 6-15. As we saw previously, in the normal situation the sodium current first increases, and then decreases after a step depolarization as the channels open and then close with a delay (see Figure 6-15A). After a protease is applied to the internal face of the membrane (see Figure 6-15B), the sodium current increases upon depolarization, as before, but now the current remains on for the duration of the depolarization: The inactivation gate has been destroyed but activation is normal. This supports the idea that there are two separate gates controlling access to the sodium channel pore. It also suggests that the inactivation gate is on the intracellular part of the channel protein molecule, because the proteolytic enzyme is ineffective on the outside of the membrane.

The Temporal Behavior of Sodium and Potassium Conductance

To specify the time course of the changes in sodium and potassium conductances following a depolarizing voltage-clamp step, it is sufficient to know the behavior of the gating parameters m, *n*, and *h*. In equation form, the sodium and potassium conductances would be given by

$$g_{Na} = \bar{g}_{Na} m^3 h \qquad (6\text{-}10)$$

$$g_K = \bar{g}_K n^4 \qquad (6\text{-}11)$$

where $\bar{g}_{Na}$ and $\bar{g}_K$ are the maximal sodium and potassium conductances, and *m*, *n*, and *h* are given by Equations (6-6), (6-8), and (6-9), respectively. Thus, following a depolarization, the sodium conductance rises in proportion to the third power of the activation parameter *m* and falls in direct proportion to the decline in the inactivation parameter *h*. The potassium conductance rises as the fourth power of its activation parameter and does not inactivate. The names used in Chapter 5 for the various voltage-sensitive gates of the potassium and sodium channels derive from the variables chosen by Hodgkin and Huxley to represent these activation and inactivation parameters. The sodium activation gate is called the *m* gate, the sodium inactivation gate the *h* gate, and the potassium gate the *n* gate, to reflect the roles of these parameters in Equations (6-10) and (6-11).

The surest test of a theory like the Hodgkin-Huxley theory of the action potential is to see if it can quantitatively describe the event it is supposed to explain. Hodgkin and Huxley tested their theory in this way by determining whether they could quantitatively reconstruct the action potential of a squid giant axon using the system of equations they derived from their analysis of voltage-clamp data. Because the action potential does not occur under voltage-clamp conditions, this required knowing both the voltage dependence and the time dependence of a large number of parameters. This included knowing how the rate constants for all three gating particles and how the maximum values of *h*, *m*, and *n* depend on the membrane voltage. All of these parameters could be determined experimentally from a complete set of voltage-clamp experiments, allowing Hodgkin and Huxley to calculate the action potential that would occur if their axon were not "voltage clamped." They then compared their calculated action potential with the action potential recorded from the same axon when the voltage-clamp apparatus was switched off. They found that the calculated action potential reproduced all the features of the real one in exquisite detail, confirming that they had covered all the relevant features of the nerve membrane involved in the generation of the action potential.

Gating Currents

Hodgkin and Huxley realized that their scheme for the gating of the sodium and potassium channel predicted that there should be an electrical current flow within the membrane associated with the movement of the charged gating particles. When a step change in membrane potential is made, the charged gating particles redistribute within the membrane; because the movement of charge through space is an electrical current (by definition), this redistribution of charges from one face of the membrane to the other should be measurable as a rapid component of membrane current in response to the voltage change. A current of this type flowing within a material is called a **displacement current**. The equipment available to Hodgkin and Huxley was inadequate to detect this small current, however. Almost 20 years later, Armstrong and Bezanilla managed to measure the displacement current associated with the movement of the gating particles.

The procedure for measuring the displacement currents, which have come to be called **gating currents** because of their presumed function in the membrane, is illustrated in Figure 6-16. The basic idea is to start by holding the membrane potential at a hyperpolarized level; this ensures that all the gating particles are on the inner face of the membrane (assuming, once again, that the gating particles are positively charged). In addition, all the sodium and potassium currents through the channels are blocked by drugs, like tetrodotoxin and TEA. A step is then made to a more hyperpolarized level, say 30 mV more negative. Because all the gating charges are already on the inner face of the membrane, no displacement current will flow as the result of this hyperpolarizing step. The only current flowing in this situation will be the rapid influx of negative charge necessary to step the voltage down. The voltage is then returned to the original hyperpolarized holding level, and a 30-mV depolarizing step is made. The influx of positive charge necessary to depolarize by 30 mV will be equal in magnitude, but opposite in sign, to the influx of negative charge necessary to make the previous 30-mV hyperpolarizing step. However, the depolarizing step will in addition cause some gating charges to move from the inner to the outer face of the membrane. Thus, there will be an extra component of current, due to the movement of gating charges, in response to the depolarizing step. By subtracting the current in response to the hyperpolarizing step from the depolarizing current, this extra gating current can be isolated. Experiments on this gating current sug-

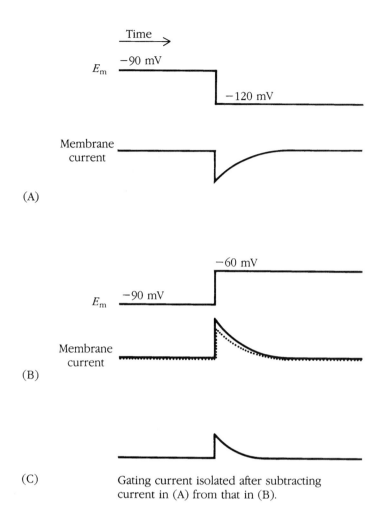

(A)

(B)

(C)

Gating current isolated after subtracting current in (A) from that in (B).

Figure 6-16
Procedure for isolating the gating current associated with the opening of voltage-sensitive sodium channels of an axon membrane. (A) The membrane voltage is stepped negative from a hyperpolarized level. With all ion channels blocked, the only current flowing is that required to move the membrane voltage more negative. (B) The membrane voltage is stepped positive from a hyperpolarized level. The current necessary to move the potential in the positive direction (dotted trace) will be the same amplitude, but opposite sign, as in (A). In addition, there will be an extra component of current in (B) caused by the movement of the charged gating particles in response to the depolarization. (C) The extra component is seen on an expanded vertical scale.

gest that it has the right voltage dependence and other properties to indeed represent the charge displacement underlying the gating scheme suggested by Hodgkin and Huxley. This is an important piece of evidence validating a basic feature of the Hodgkin-Huxley model of the membrane of excitable cells.

Summary

Hodgkin and Huxley made the fundamental observations on which our current understanding of the ionic basis of the action potential is based. In their experiments, they measured the ionic currents flowing across the membrane of a squid giant axon in response to changes in membrane voltage. This was done using the voltage-clamp apparatus, which provides a means of holding the membrane potential constant in the face of changes in the ionic conductance of the axon membrane. By analyzing these ionic currents, Hodgkin and Huxley derived equations specifying both the voltage dependence and the time course of changes in sodium and potassium conductance of the membrane. During a maintained depolarization, the sodium conductance increased rapidly and then declined, while potassium conductance showed a delayed but maintained increase. Analysis of the change in sodium conductance suggested that the conducting state of the sodium channel was controlled by a rapidly opening activation gate, called the *m* gate, and a slowly closing inactivation gate, called the *h* gate. The gates behave as though they are controlled by charged gating particles that move within the plasma membrane; when the gating particles occupy binding sites associated with the channel gating mechanism, the gates open. The kinetics of the observed gating behavior would be explained by the kinetics of the redistribution of the charged gating particles within the membrane following a step change in the transmembrane potential. The sodium activation gate appears to open when three independent binding sites are occupied by gating particles, while the inactivation gate closes when a single particle leaves a single binding site. The potassium channel is controlled by a single gate, the *n* gate, which opens when four binding sites are occupied. The rate at which the gating particles redistribute following a depolarization is different for the three types of gate, with sodium activation gating being faster than sodium inactivation or potassium activation. Tiny membrane currents associated with the movement of the charged gating particles within the membrane have been detected. Experiments combining molecular biology with electrical measurements promise to establish the correspondence between Hodgkin and Huxley's gating mechanisms and actual parts of the ion channel protein molecule.

Synaptic Transmission at the Neuromuscular Junction

Chapter 5 was concerned with the ionic basis of the action potential, the electrical signal that carries messages long distances along nerve fibers. Using the patellar reflex as an example, we discussed the mechanism that allows the message that the muscle was stretched to travel along the membrane of the sensory neuron from the sensory endings in the muscle to the termination of the sensory fiber in the spinal cord. After the message is passed to the motor neuron within the spinal cord, action potentials also carry the electrical signal back down the nerve to the muscle, to activate the reflexive contraction of the muscle. This chapter is concerned with the mechanism by which action potential activity in the motor neuron can be passed along to the cells of the muscle, causing the muscle cells to contract. In Chapter 8, we discuss how action potentials in the sensory neuron influence the activity of the motor neuron in the spinal cord.

Chemical and Electrical Synapses

The point where activity is transmitted from one nerve cell to another or from a motor neuron to a muscle cell is called a **synapse**. In the patellar reflex, there are two synapses: the one between the sensory neuron and the motor neuron in the spinal cord, and the one between the motor neuron and the cells of the quadriceps muscle. There are two general classes of synapses: electrical synapses and chemical synapses. In both types, there are specialized membrane structures at the point where the input cell, called the **presynaptic cell**, comes into contact with the output cell, called the **postsynaptic cell**.

At a chemical synapse, an action potential in the presynaptic cell causes it to release a chemical substance (called a **neurotransmitter**) that diffuses through the extracellular space and changes the membrane potential of the postsynaptic cell. At an electrical synapse, part of a change in membrane potential (such as the depolarization during an action potential) in the presynaptic cell spreads directly to the postsynaptic cell without the action of any intermediary chemical. Both synapses in the patellar reflex, and indeed most synapses in mammalian nervous systems, are chemical synapses. At a chemical synapse, the membranes of the presynaptic and postsynaptic cells come close to each other but are still separated by a small gap of extracellular space. At an electrical synapse, the presynaptic and postsynaptic membranes touch and the cell interiors are directly interconnected by means of special ion channels called gap junctions that allow electrical current to flow from one cell to another. In this chapter we concentrate on chemical synaptic transmission. Electrical synaptic transmission is described in more detail in Chapter 11.

The Neuromuscular Junction as a Model Chemical Synapse

The best understood chemical synapse is that between a motor neuron and a muscle cell. This synapse is given the special name **neuromuscular junction** (also sometimes called the **myoneural junction**). Although the fine details may differ somewhat, the basic scheme that describes the functioning of the neuromuscular junction applies to all chemical synapses, as far as is known. Therefore, this chapter concentrates on the characteristics of this special synapse at the end of the patellar reflex. In the next chapter, we consider some of the differences between the synapse at the neuromuscular junction and synapses in the central nervous system, like the synapse between the sensory and motor neurons in the spinal cord.

Transmission at a Chemical Synapse

The sequence of events during neuromuscular synaptic transmission is summarized in Figure 7-1. When an action potential arrives

1. Presynaptic action potential

↓

2. Depolarization of synaptic terminal

↓

3. Release of chemical neurotransmitter molecules

↓

4. Neurotransmitter molecules bind to special receptors on postsynaptic cell

↓

5. Change in ionic permeability of postsynaptic cell

↓

6. Change in membrane potential of postsynaptic cell

Figure 7-1
Sequence of events during transmission at a chemical synapse.

Figure 7-2
Chemical structure of acetylcholine (ACh), the chemical neurotransmitter at the neuromuscular junction.

at the end of the motor neuron nerve fiber, it invades a specialized structure called the **synaptic terminal**. Depolarization of the synaptic terminal induces release of a chemical messenger that is stored inside the terminal. At the vertebrate neuromuscular junction, this chemical messenger is **acetylcholine** (abbreviated ACh), whose chemical structure is shown in Figure 7-2. ACh diffuses across the space separating the presynaptic motor neuron terminal from the postsynaptic muscle cell and alters the ionic permeability of the muscle cell membrane. The change in ionic permeability produces a depolarization of the muscle cell membrane. The remainder of this chapter describes in detail this basic sequence of events.

Presynaptic Action Potential and Acetylcholine Release

The occurrence of an action potential in the synaptic terminal is the trigger for ACh release. It has been demonstrated that the de-

Figure 7-3
Sequence of events between the arrival of an action potential at a synaptic terminal and the release of chemical transmitter.

1. Presynaptic action potential

2. Depolarization of synaptic terminal

3. Voltage-sensitive calcium channels open

4. Calcium enters synaptic terminal

5. Release of chemical neurotransmitter

polarization during the action potential is the necessary stimulus for transmitter release; any experimental manipulation that depolarizes the synaptic terminal causes ACh to be released. This coupling between depolarization and release is not direct, however. The signal that mediates this coupling is the influx into the synaptic terminal of ions in the ECF that we have largely ignored to this point—calcium ions.

Calcium is present at low concentration in ECF (1–2 mM) and is not important in resting membrane potentials or in most nerve action potentials, although calcium influx contributes to some action potentials (see Chapter 5). However, calcium ions must be present in the ECF in order for release of chemical neurotransmitter to occur. If calcium ions are removed from the ECF, depolarization of the synaptic terminal can no longer induce the release of ACh. Thus, depolarization causes external calcium ions to enter the synaptic terminal, and the calcium in turn causes ACh to be released from the terminal.

What mechanism underlies the linkage between depolarization of the terminal and influx of calcium ions? As we've seen in earlier chapters, ions cross membranes through specialized transmembrane channels, and calcium ions are no different in this regard. The membrane of the synaptic terminal contains calcium channels that are closed as long as E_m is near its normal resting level. These channels are similar in behavior to the voltage-dependent potassium channels of nerve membrane; they open upon depolarization and close again when the membrane potential repolarizes. Thus, when an action potential invades the synaptic terminal, the calcium permeability of the membrane increases during the depolarizing phase of the action potential and declines again as membrane potential returns to normal.

Although the external calcium concentration is small (1–2 mM), the internal concentration of calcium ions that are free to diffuse across the plasma membrane is much smaller ($< 10^{-6}$ M). From the Nernst equation, then, the equilibrium potential for calcium would be expected to be positive. Therefore, both the concentration and the electrical gradients for calcium drive calcium into the terminal, and when calcium permeability increases, there will be an influx of calcium. During a presynaptic action potential, there is a spike of calcium entry into the terminal, resulting in a release of neurotransmitter into the extracellular space. This sequence is summarized in Figure 7-3.

Effect of Acetylcholine on the Muscle Cell

The goal of synaptic transmission at the neuromuscular junction is to cause the muscle cell to contract. ACh released from the synaptic terminal accomplishes this goal by depolarizing the muscle cell. Because muscle cells are excitable cells like neurons, this depolarization will set in motion an all-or-none propagating action potential if the depolarization exceeds threshold. The coupling between the muscle action potential and contraction is the subject of Chapter 9. This section discusses the effect of ACh on the muscle cell membrane.

The region of muscle membrane where synaptic contact is made is called the **end-plate** region, and it possesses special characteristics. In particular, the end-plate membrane is rich in a transmembrane protein that acts as an ionic channel. Unlike the voltage-dependent channels discussed in Chapter 5, however, this channel is little affected by membrane potential. Instead, this channel is sensitive to ACh: It opens when it binds ACh. Thus, ACh released from the synaptic terminal diffuses across the synaptic cleft to the muscle membrane, where it combines with specific receptors associated with the ionic channel. As shown schematically in Figure 7-4, the gate on the channel is closed in the absence of ACh. When the receptor sites are occupied, however, the protein undergoes a conformational change, the gate opens, and the channel allows ions across the membrane. Current evidence indicates that two ACh molecules must bind to the chan-

Figure 7-4

Schematic representation of the behavior of the ACh-sensitive channel in the end-plate membrane. When two molecules of ACh are bound to the ACh binding sites of the channel, the gate opens, allowing sodium and potassium ions to flow through the channel.

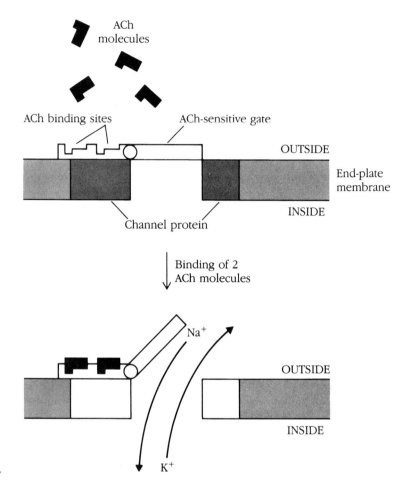

Figure 7-5

Opening a channel that allows both potassium and sodium to cross the membrane results in a higher value for p_{Na}/p_K and causes depolarization.

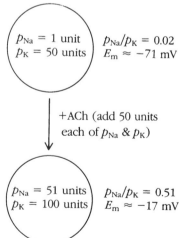

nel in order for the gate to open. The ACh-binding site is highly specific; only ACh or a small number of structurally related compounds can bind to the site and cause the channel to open.

The ACh-activated channel of the muscle end-plate allows both sodium and potassium to cross the membrane about equally well. Thus, when ACh is present, the membrane permeability to both sodium and potassium increases. How can such an increase in permeability produce a depolarization of the muscle cell? To see this, consider the situation diagrammed in Figure 7-5. Recall from Chapter 4 that membrane potential depends on the relative sodium and potassium permeabilities of the membrane (the Goldman equation). For the cell of Figure 7-5, p_{Na}/p_K is 0.02 at rest and E_m would be about -71 mV, assuming typical ECF and ICF (see Table 1-1). In the presence of ACh, however, p_{Na} and p_K increase by equal amounts; p_{Na}/p_K increases to 0.51 and E_m depolarizes to about -17 mV.

In a muscle cell, the situation is somewhat more complicated than that depicted in Figure 7-5 because the ACh-activated channels are spatially restricted to the end-plate region. Thus, the increase in permeability occurs in only part of the cell membrane. In such a situation, the result would be quantitatively different from but qualitatively similar to the example in Figure 7-5.

The ACh-activated channels are packed densely in the muscle end-plate region, and this provides a good opportunity to visualize the protein molecules that form the channel. Because the protein molecules are very small, however, it is only at high power under the electron microscope that the ACh receptor and its channel can be discerned. A picture of a postsynaptic membrane examined in this way is shown in Figure 7-6. The membrane is studded with ring-shaped particles that are found only at the region of synaptic contact. These particles have been isolated from the postsynaptic membrane and chemically identified as the ACh-binding receptor molecule and its associated channel. The hole in the middle is probably the aqueous pore through which the sodium and potassium ions cross the membrane. The ACh-activated channels have been chemically isolated from muscle membrane, and can be inserted into artificial membranes as in Figure 7-6B. The molecular structure of the ACh-activated channel will be described in more detail later in this chapter.

Neurotransmitter Release

We now return to the synaptic terminal for a more detailed examination of the mechanism of neurotransmitter release. ACh is released from the motor nerve terminal in quanta consisting of many molecules. Thus, the basic unit of release is not a single molecule of ACh, but the quantum. At the neuromuscular junction, it is estimated that a single quantum of ACh contains about 10,000 molecules. An individual quantum is either released all together or not released at all. The release of ACh during neuromuscular transmission can be thought of as the sudden appearance of a "puff" of ACh molecules in the extracellular space as the entire content of a quantum is released. A single presynaptic action potential normally causes the release of more than a hundred quanta from the synaptic terminal.

The original suggestion that ACh is released in multimolecular

0.1 μm

A

50 nm

B

Figure 7-6
(A) A view through the electron microscope at the face of the postsynaptic membrane of the electric organ of the electrical skate, *Torpedo*. This organ, which is a rich source of ACh receptors for biochemical study, is a specialized type of muscle tissue. The membrane particles are the ACh-activated channels of the postsynaptic membrane. (B) Several views of individual ACh receptors that have been chemically isolated from preparations like that in (A), then placed in artificial membranes. (Courtesy of J. Cartaud of the Institut Jacques Monod, CNRS/Université Paris 7, France.)

(A)

(B)

Figure 7-7
Quantized responses of muscle cell to action potentials in the presynaptic motor neuron. The arrows indicate the timing of the presynaptic action potentials. (B) The graph shows the peak response amplitudes that might be recorded in response to a series of several hundred presynaptic action potentials as in (A).

quanta was made on the basis of a statistical analysis of the response of the postsynaptic muscle cell to action potentials in the presynaptic motor neuron. This analysis was first carried out by P. Fatt and B. Katz, and it initiated a series of studies by Katz and co-workers that gave rise to the basic scheme for chemical neurotransmission presented in this chapter. Experimentally, the analysis was accomplished by reducing the extracellular calcium concentration to the point where the influx of calcium ions into the synaptic terminal during an action potential was much less than usual. Under these conditions, a single presynaptic action potential released on average only one or two quanta of ACh instead of more than a hundred. Examples of end-plate potentials recorded in a muscle cell in response to a series of presynaptic action potentials are shown in Figure 7-7. Because only a small number of quanta are released per action potential, the end-plate potentials in the reduced-calcium ECF are much smaller than usual and do not reach threshold for generating an action potential in the muscle cell. Notice that the amplitude of the depolarization of the muscle cell fluctuates considerably over the series of presynaptic action potentials: Sometimes there was a large response and other times there was no response at all. Fatt and Katz measured a large number of such

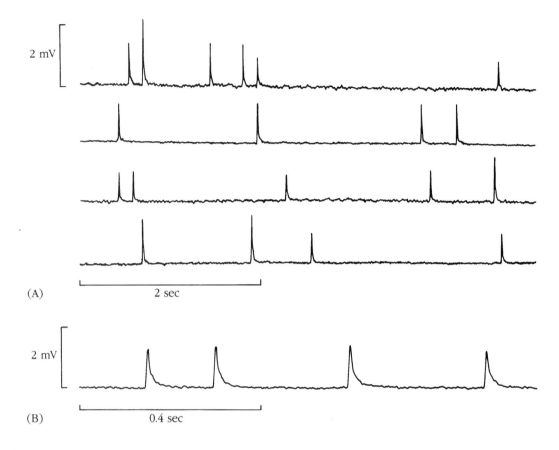

(A)

2 sec

(B)

0.4 sec

2 mV

2 mV

Figure 7-8
Spontaneous miniature end-plate potentials recorded from the end-plate region of a muscle cell. These randomly occurring small depolarizations of the muscle cell are caused by the spontaneous release of single quanta of ACh from the synaptic terminal of the motor neuron. (A) Four 5-second samples of muscle cell E_m, measured via an intracellular microelectrode. The spontaneous depolarizations occur at a rate of approximately one per second. (B) Spontaneous miniature end-plate potentials viewed on an expanded time scale to show the shape of the events more clearly. (Unpublished data from G. Matthews)

responses and found that the amplitudes clustered around particular values that were integral multiples of the smallest observed response. For example, as shown in Figure 7-7B, there might be a cluster of responses that were 1 mV in amplitude, another cluster at 2 mV, and another at 3 mV. This indicates that the response was quantized in irreducible units of 1 mV, and that the presynaptic action potential released ACh in corresponding quantal units. Thus, a given presynaptic action potential might cause the release of three, two, one, or no quanta, but not 0.5 or 1.5 quanta.

Fatt and Katz also observed that there were occasional, small depolarizations that occurred in the absence of any presynaptic action potential. They noted that these spontaneous depolarizations always had the same amplitude as the single quantum response produced by a presynaptic action potential in low-calcium ECF. That is, if the irreducible unit of evoked muscle response was 1 mV, then the spontaneous events also were about 1 mV in amplitude. Figure 7-8 shows several of these spontaneous depolarizations recorded inside a muscle cell. These events are called miniature end-plate potentials, and are assumed to result from the spontaneous release of single quanta of ACh from the synaptic terminal. Under normal conditions, these spontaneous events occur at a low rate—about one or two per second; however, any manipulation that depolarizes the nerve terminal increases their rate of occurrence, confirming that their source is the process that couples depolarization to quantal ACh release during the normal functioning of the nerve terminal.

The Vesicle Hypothesis of Quantal Transmitter Release

To understand the basis of the packaging of ACh in quanta, it is necessary to look at the structure of the synaptic terminal, which is shown schematically in Figure 7-9. The terminal contains a large number of tiny, membrane-bound structures called **synaptic vesicles**. These vesicles contain ACh, and it is natural to assume that they represent the packets of ACh that are released in response to a presynaptic action potential. Indeed, these vesicles are depleted by any manipulation, such as prolonged depolarization or firing of large numbers of action potentials, which causes release of large amounts of ACh. It is now generally accepted that release of ACh is accomplished by the fusion of the vesicle membrane with the plasma membrane of the terminal, so that the contents of the vesicle are dumped into the extracellular space between the terminal and the muscle cell. The vesicles do not fuse with the plasma membrane just anywhere; rather, they apparently fuse only at specialized membrane regions, called **release sites** or **active zones**, that are found only on the membrane face opposite the postsynaptic muscle cell. Thus, quanta of ACh are released only into the narrow space, the **synaptic cleft**, separating the presynaptic and postsynaptic cells. A close-up, schematic view of the fusion of a synaptic vesicle with the plasma membrane is shown in Figure 7-10. With freeze-fracture electron microscopy, the active zone of the presynaptic terminal appears as a double row of large membrane particles, which are probably membrane proteins involved in the fusion between the membrane of the synaptic vesicle and the presynaptic plasma membrane. Examples of these active zone particles can be seen in Figure 7-11.

Elegant evidence for vesicle fusion as the mechanism of ACh release was provided by anatomical experiments by Heuser, Reese,

Figure 7-9
The structure of the region of synaptic contact at the neuromuscular junction.

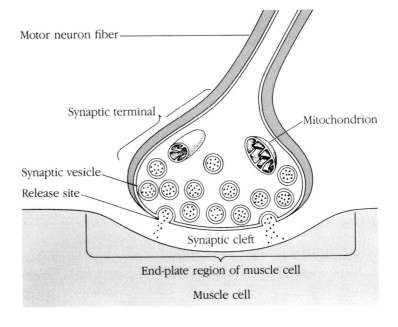

Figure 7-10
Close-up view of the synaptic region during the release of ACh at the neuromuscular junction.

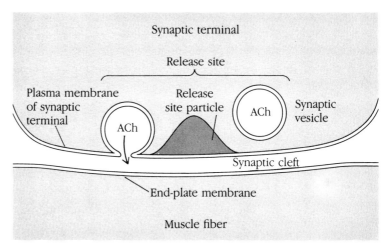

Dennis, Jan, Jan, and Evans. In these experiments, a muscle and its attached nerve were placed in an apparatus that could very rapidly freeze the nerve and muscle. Heuser and his co-workers then literally froze the release process at the instant just after arrival of an action potential in the synaptic terminal and examined the frozen tissue in the electron microscope, using the freeze-fracture technique discussed in Chapter 1. They saw what appeared to be synaptic vesicles in the process of fusing with the plasma membrane,

A   B

Figure 7-11

Electron micrographs of the freeze-fractured face of a presynaptic terminal at the neuromuscular junction. (A) An unstimulated nerve terminal. Note the double row of particles defining a presynaptic release site or active zone (az). The arrow points to what appears to be a synaptic vesicle spontaneously fusing with the presynaptic membrane. Such spontaneous fusions presumably underlie the spontaneous miniature end-plate potentials shown in Figure 7-8. The arrowhead at the left points to a synaptic vesicle visible in a region where the membrane fractured all the way through to reveal a portion of the intracellular fluid. (B) A higher-power view of an active zone of a nerve terminal frozen during the release of ACh stimulated by presynaptic action potentials. The ice-filled depressions arrayed along either side of the active zone correspond to regions where synaptic vesicles are in the process of fusing with the presynaptic membrane. (Reproduced from Ko C.-P. Regeneration of the active zone at the frog neuromuscular junction. *Cell Biol* 1984;98:1685–1695 by copyright permission of the Rockefeller University Press.)

as shown in Figure 7-11. The fusing vesicles appeared as ice-filled pits or depressions in the presynaptic membrane, lined up along the presynaptic release sites. They saw such fusion only when ACh release should have been occurring, not before or after the action potential in the terminal. Further, the fusion occurred only when calcium was present in the ECF, which as we know is prerequisite for release to occur.

One of the great remaining mysteries in the mechanism of synaptic transmission is the linkage between calcium entry and vesicle fusion. No one yet understands how an increase in internal calcium increases the probability that a vesicle will fuse with the plasma membrane of the synaptic terminal. It is likely that there are calcium-binding molecules associated with the release sites and with the vesicle membrane and that binding of calcium somehow alters the interactions among these molecules. The rows of membrane particles seen in freeze-fracture views of the presynaptic release sites (see Figure 7-11) may correspond to these molecules that regulate the interaction between the vesicles and the presynaptic membrane. However, the molecular mechanism remains unknown.

Recycling of Vesicle Membrane

If the membranes of synaptic vesicles fused with the plasma membrane of the terminal during transmitter release, we might expect the area of the terminal membrane to increase with use. Indeed, over the life span of an animal, millions of synaptic vesicles might fuse with the terminal membrane, so that the terminal might become huge. However, this does not happen because the vesicle membrane does not remain part of the plasma membrane; instead, Heuser and Reese found that the fused vesicles are recycled. The scheme is summarized in Figure 7-12. After fusion, the vesicles pinch off again from the plasma membrane, are refilled with ACh, and are ready to be used again to transfer neurotransmitter into the synaptic cleft.

Inactivation of Released Acetylcholine

We have seen how ACh is released from the synaptic terminal and how it depolarizes the postsynaptic muscle cell. How is the action of ACh terminated so that the end-plate region returns to its

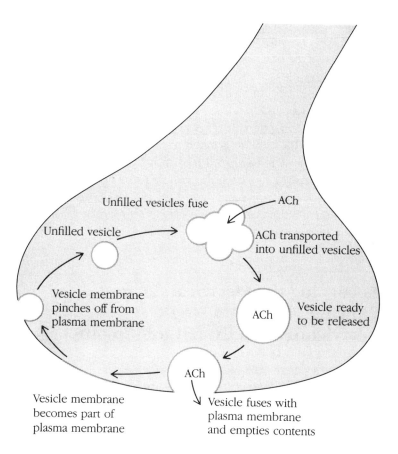

Figure 7-12
The recycling of vesicle membrane in the presynaptic terminal at the neuromuscular junction. The vesicle membrane is shown in gray and the plasma membrane in black.

Unfilled vesicles fuse

ACh

Unfilled vesicle

ACh transported into unfilled vesicles

Vesicle membrane pinches off from plasma membrane

ACh

Vesicle ready to be released

ACh

Vesicle membrane becomes part of plasma membrane

ACh

Vesicle fuses with plasma membrane and empties contents

resting state? The answer is that there is another specialized ACh binding protein in the end-plate region. This protein is the enzyme acetylcholinesterase, which splits ACh into acetate and choline. Because neither acetate nor choline can bind to and activate the ACh-activated channel, acetylcholinesterase effectively halts the action of any ACh it encounters.

When a puff of ACh is released in response to an action potential in the synaptic terminal, the concentration of ACh in the synaptic cleft abruptly rises. Some of the released ACh molecules will bind to ACh-activated channels, causing them to open and increasing the sodium and potassium permeability of the end-plate membrane; other ACh molecules will bind to acetylcholinesterase and be inactivated. Even though the binding of ACh to the postsynaptic channel is highly specific, it is readily reversible; the binding typically lasts for only about 1 msec. When an ACh molecule comes off a gate, the channel closes. The newly freed ACh molecule may then bind again to an ACh-activated channel, or it might bind to acetylcholinesterase and be inactivated. With time following release of the puff, the concentration of ACh in the cleft will fall until all of the released ACh has been split into acetate and choline.

It would be wasteful if the choline resulting from inactivation of ACh were lost and had to be replaced with fresh choline from inside the presynaptic cell. This potential waste is avoided because most of the choline is taken back up into the synaptic terminal, where it is reassembled into ACh by the enzyme choline acetyltransferase. Thus, both the vesicle membrane (the packaging material of the quantum) and the released neurotransmitter (the contents of the quantum) are effectively recycled by the presynaptic terminal.

Recording the Electrical Current Flowing Through a Single Acetylcholine-Activated Ion Channel

Throughout our discussion of the membrane properties of excitable cells, we have made extensive use of the notion of ions crossing the membrane through specific pores or channels. For example, we saw that the effect of ACh on the muscle membrane is mediated via ion channels in the postsynaptic membrane that open in the presence of ACh. As discussed in Chapters 4 and 6, the flow of ions across the cell membrane constitutes a transmembrane electrical current that can be measured with electrical techniques like the voltage clamp. Recently, a new technique was developed by Neher and Sakmann to record transmembrane ionic currents, and the technique has sufficient resolution to measure the minute electrical current flowing through a single open ion channel. The technique is called the **patch clamp**, and it is illustrated in Figure 7-13.

The basic idea behind the patch clamp is to isolate electrically a small patch of cell membrane that contains only a few ionic channels. The electrical isolation is achieved by placing a specially constructed miniature glass pipette in close contact with the membrane, so that a tight seal forms between the membrane and the glass. When one of the ion channels in the isolated patch opens, electrical current flows across the membrane; in the case of the ACh-activated channel that current would be a net inward (that is, depolarizing) current under normal conditions. We know

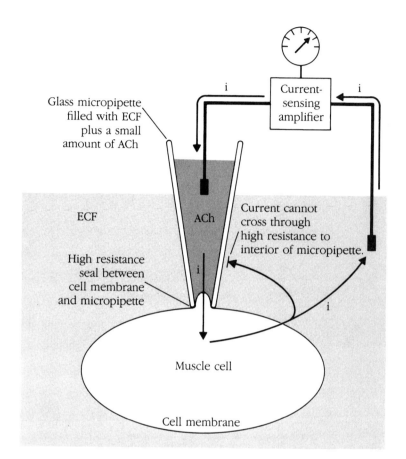

Figure 7-13
Schematic illustration of the procedure for recording the current through a single ACh-activated channel in a cell membrane. A micropipette with a tip diameter of 1 to 2 mm is placed on the external surface of the membrane. A tight electrical seal is made between the membrane and the glass of the micropipette, so that a resistance greater than 10^{10} ohms is imposed in the extracellular path for current flow through the channel. When a channel in the patch of membrane inside the micropipette opens, a current-sensing amplifier connected to the interior of the pipette detects the minute current flow.

from the basic properties of electricity that current must flow in a complete circuit. As shown in Figure 7-13, the return current path through the extracellular space is broken by the presence of the glass pipette; there is a high electrical resistance imposed by the seal between the cell membrane and the pipette. Under these conditions, the ionic current through the open channel is forced to complete its circuit through the current-sensing amplifier connected to the interior of the pipette. In order for the patch-clamp technique to achieve sufficient sensitivity to measure the current through a single channel, the electrical resistance between the interior of the patch pipette and the extracellular space must be greater than about 10^9 ohms, which is a very large resistance indeed. Fortunately for neurophysiologists, it is possible to achieve resistances greater than 10^{10} ohms.

Using the patch clamp, it is possible to record the current through ACh-activated channels of the postsynaptic membrane of muscle

Figure 7-14
(A) The current that would be expected to flow through a single ACh-activated channel if the conducting state of the channel is controlled by a single gate that is either open all the way or closed all the way. When ACh binds to the gating portion of the channel, the channel opens and there is a stepwise pulse of inward current flowing through the channel. When ACh unbinds, the channel closes and the current abruptly disappears. (B) Actual recordings of currents flowing through single ACh-activated channels of human muscle cells maintained in cell culture. Note that at the asterisk two channels opened simultaneously, and their currents added independently. These recordings show the fundamental postsynaptic events that underlie the interaction between the nervous system and the muscles in the human body. (Reproduced with permission from Jackson MB, Lecar H, Askanas V, Engel WK. Single cholinergic receptor channel currents in cultured human muscle. *J. Neurosci* 1982;2:1465–1473.)

(A)

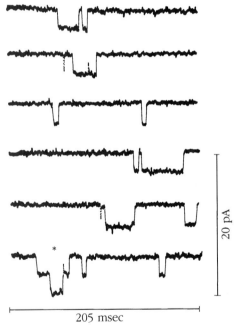

(B)   Actual Recordings from Jackson *et al.*

cells by placing a small amount of ACh (or structurally related compounds that are recognized by the receptors on the gate) inside the patch pipette. As shown in Figure 7-4, when the receptors are occupied, the gate opens and the channel allows ions to cross the membrane. Schematically, then, we might expect to record an electrical current like that shown in Figure 7-14A when the channel opens. There would be a rapid step of inward current that occurs as the gate opens, the current would be maintained at a constant level for as long as the channel is open, and the step would terminate when ACh unbinds from one of the receptor sites, causing the gate to close. If a second channel opens while the first is still open, the two currents simply add to produce a current twice as large as the single-channel current. This is also shown in Figure 7-14A.

Actual patch-clamp recordings of currents through single ACh-activated channels of human muscle cells are shown in Figure 7-14B. These records show that the currents through the channels are the rectangular events expected from the simple gating scheme of Figure 7-4. Experiments like that of Figure 7-14B confirm directly the view of ion permeation and channel gating that we have used to explain the electrical behavior of the membranes of excitable cells: The gated ion channels carrying electrical current across the plasma membrane are not just figments of the neurophysiologist's imagination. The development of the patch-clamp technique has led to a flurry of new information about ion channels of all types; for example, the voltage-sensitive sodium and potassium channels that underlie the action potential (see Chapters 5 and 6) have also been studied using this technique.

Molecular Properties of the Acetylcholine-Activated Channel

Techniques of molecular biology are being applied with great success to the study of ion channel function, particularly when combined with measurements of single-channel behavior using the patch-clamp technique just described. This has been especially true for the ACh-activated channel of the muscle end-plate. Biochemical studies have shown that this channel is formed by the aggregation of five individual protein subunits: two copies of an α-subunit, plus β-, γ-, and δ-subunits. The two ACh-binding sites have been located, one on each of the two α-subunits, thus accounting neatly for the fact that binding of two ACh molecules is required to open the channel (see Figure 7-4). The subunits come together as shown in Figure 7-15 to form the ACh-activated channel, with parts of each subunit forming the aqueous pore at the center through which cations can cross the membrane. The genes encoding each of these subunits have been identified and analyzed, and the sequence of amino acids making up the protein has been deduced in each case by reading the genetic code

Figure 7-15
Molecular structure of the ACh-activated channel, shown from the side and from above. The five subunits interact as shown to form the gated ion channel of the end-plate membrane.

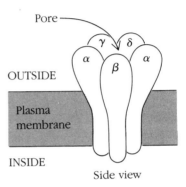

from the pattern of nucleic acids in the DNA. This sequence of amino acids gives valuable structural information about the ACh-activated channel. Beyond that, molecular biological techniques can be used to assign functional roles to particular parts of the channel protein. This approach makes use of the fact that it is possible to make messenger RNA (mRNA) from the DNA sequence of the channel protein; when this mRNA is injected into a cell that does not normally make ACh-activated channels (such as the egg cell of a frog), the cell's machinery of protein synthesis will read the message and make functional ACh-activated channels. The properties of these channels can then be examined using patch-clamp recording. Thus, by altering the mRNA, experimenters can make discrete changes in the channel protein and then see how the change affects the behavior of the channel. For example, in this way the parts of each subunit that probably make up the ion-conducting pore have been identified.

Summary

The sequence of events during synaptic transmission at the neuromuscular junction is summarized in Figure 7-16. The depolariza-

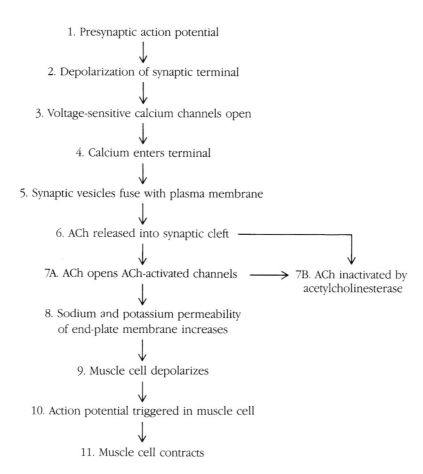

1. Presynaptic action potential
   ↓
2. Depolarization of synaptic terminal
   ↓
3. Voltage-sensitive calcium channels open
   ↓
4. Calcium enters terminal
   ↓
5. Synaptic vesicles fuse with plasma membrane
   ↓
6. ACh released into synaptic cleft ────────────┐
   ↓   ↓
7A. ACh opens ACh-activated channels ──────→ 7B. ACh inactivated by
   ↓   acetylcholinesterase
8. Sodium and potassium permeability
   of end-plate membrane increases
   ↓
9. Muscle cell depolarizes
   ↓
10. Action potential triggered in muscle cell
   ↓
11. Muscle cell contracts

Figure 7-16
Summary of the sequence of events during synaptic transmission at the neuromuscular junction.

tion produced by an action potential in the synaptic terminal opens voltage-dependent calcium channels in the terminal membrane. Calcium ions enter the terminal down their concentration and electrical gradients, inducing synaptic vesicles filled with ACh to fuse with the plasma membrane facing the muscle cell. The ACh is thereby dumped into the synaptic cleft, and some of it diffuses to the muscle membrane and combines with specific receptors on ACh-activated channels in the muscle membrane. When ACh is bound, the channel opens and allows sodium and potassium ions to cross the membrane. This depolarizes the muscle membrane and triggers an all-or-none action potential in the muscle cell. The action of ACh is terminated by the enzyme acetylcholinesterase, which splits ACh into acetate and choline.

Synaptic Transmission in the Central Nervous System

Chemical synapses between neurons operate according to the same general principles as the synapse between a motor neuron and a muscle cell discussed in the previous chapter. Thus, in the patellar reflex, an action potential in the sensory neuron depolarizes the quadriceps motor neuron through a sequence of events similar to that at the neuromuscular junction. There are, however, some major differences between neuron-to-neuron synapses and the neuron-to-muscle synapse discussed previously. This chapter considers some of these differences, again with specific reference to the patellar reflex.

Excitatory and Inhibitory Synapses

At the neuromuscular junction, acetylcholine depolarizes the muscle cell, causing it to fire an action potential. Synapses of this type are called **excitatory synapses** because the neurotransmitter brings the membrane potential of the postsynaptic cell toward the threshold for firing an action potential and thus tends to "excite" the postsynaptic cell. The synapse between the sensory neuron and the quadriceps motor neuron in the patellar reflex is an example of an excitatory synapse between two neurons. Synapses between neurons are not always excitatory, however. At **inhibitory synapses,** the neurotransmitter acts to keep the membrane potential of the postsynaptic cell more negative than the threshold potential; because this tends to prevent the postsynaptic neuron from firing an action potential, the postsynaptic cell is "inhib-

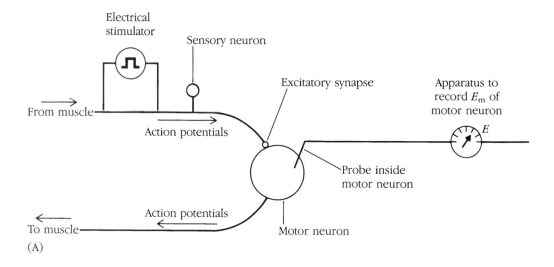

(A)

Figure 8-1

Synaptic transmission at an excitatory synapse between two neurons. (A) Experimental arrangement for examining transmission between a sensory and a motor neuron in the patellar reflex loop. (B) Responses of the postsynaptic motor neuron to action potentials in the presynaptic sensory neuron. At the upward arrows, action potentials are triggered in the presynaptic neuron by an electrical stimulus.

ited" by the release of the inhibitory neurotransmitter. The fact that not all synapses in the nervous system are excitatory is one major difference between synaptic transmission at the neuromuscular junction and synaptic transmission in the nervous system in general.

We will return to a discussion of inhibitory synapses later in this chapter. At this point, the discussion centers on the properties of excitatory synaptic transmission between neurons in the nervous system.

Excitatory Synaptic Transmission Between Neurons

The synapse at the neuromuscular junction is unusual in one important regard: A single action potential in the presynaptic motor neuron produces a sufficiently large depolarization in the postsynaptic muscle cell to trigger a postsynaptic action potential. Such a synapse is called a one-for-one synapse because one action potential appears in the output cell for each action potential in the input cell. Most synapses between neurons are not this strong. Instead, a single presynaptic action potential typically produces only a small depolarization of the postsynaptic cell. The synapse between a single stretch receptor sensory neuron and a quadriceps motor neuron is typical of this situation, and the behavior of this synapse is illustrated in Figure 8-1.

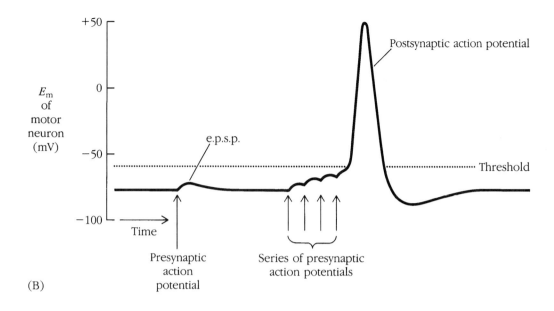

(B)

Temporal and Spatial Summation of Synaptic Potentials

Figure 8-1A shows an experimental arrangement for recording the change in membrane potential of a motor neuron when a single presynaptic sensory neuron is stimulated to fire an action potential. In this case, an intracellular probe is placed inside the sensory fiber so that an action potential can be triggered by passing a depolarizing current into the nerve fiber. Figure 8-1B shows sample results when a single action potential is triggered in the sensory neuron and when four action potentials are triggered in rapid sequence. A single presynaptic action potential produces only a small depolarizing change in the motor neuron's membrane potential. This unitary response to a presynaptic action potential is called an **excitatory postsynaptic potential (e.p.s.p.)**. A single e.p.s.p. is typically much too small to reach threshold for triggering an action potential, which usually requires a depolarization of 10 to 15 mV from the resting E_m. Figure 8-2 shows an actual recording of an e.p.s.p. in a motor neuron after a single action potential is triggered in a sensory neuron. In this experiment, an intracellular electrode was placed inside the sensory fiber to record the presynaptic membrane potential and to inject depolarizing current to elicit an action potential in the presynaptic fiber (upper recording trace). A second intracellular electrode was

E_m of sensory fiber

40 mV

E_m of motor neuron

1 mV

0.5 msec

Figure 8-2

Simultaneous intracellular recordings from a single stretch-sensitive sensory nerve fiber and a motor neuron receiving synaptic input from the sensory fiber. An action potential was triggered in the sensory fiber by passing a depolarizing electrical current through the intracellular electrode. After a brief delay, there was a small excitatory postsynaptic potential evoked in the postsynaptic motor neuron. (Unpublished data kindly provided by W. Collins, M. Honig, and L. M. Mendell of the State University of New York at Stony Brook.)

placed in the motor neuron to record the change in membrane potential of the postsynaptic cell, as diagrammed in Figure 8-1A.

If a second action potential arrives at the presynaptic terminal before the postsynaptic effect of a first action potential has disappeared, the second e.p.s.p. will sum with the first to produce a larger peak postsynaptic depolarization. As shown in Figure 8-1B, if a series of action potentials arrive in the presynaptic terminal sufficiently rapidly, it is possible for the individual e.p.s.p.'s to add up to a depolarization that reaches threshold. This kind of summation of sequential postsynaptic effects of an individual presynaptic input is called **temporal summation**. This is an important mechanism by which even a weak excitatory synaptic input can cause a neuron to fire an action potential. Figure 8-3 shows actual recordings illustrating temporal summation of e.p.s.p.'s in two different neurons. Each set of traces shows superimposed responses to three presynaptic stimuli. In each case, one stimulus fails to activate the presynaptic input and so produces no postsynaptic response (trace a), one stimulus produces a postsynaptic response that fails to reach threshold (trace b), and one stimulus produces a postsynaptic response that reaches threshold and triggers a postsynaptic action potential (trace c). Only if the successive e.p.s.p.'s summate sufficiently to reach threshold is an action potential triggered in the postsynaptic cell.

Another way that e.p.s.p.'s can sum to reach threshold is for several presynaptic neurons to fire action potentials simultaneously. In reality, a single neuron (such as the motor neuron in Figure 8-1) in the nervous system receives synaptic inputs from hundreds or even thousands of presynaptic neurons. In the patellar reflex, for example, a single quadriceps motor neuron will receive excitatory synaptic connections from many stretch receptor sensory neurons. A simplified picture of this situation is shown in Figure 8-4A. A single action potential in any one of the presynaptic

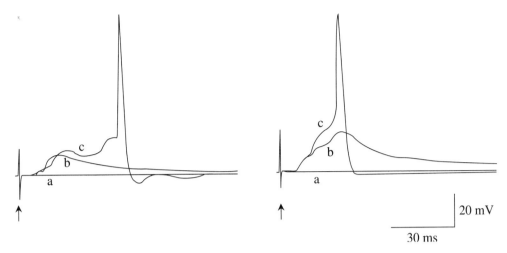

20 mV

30 ms

Figure 8-3

Intracellular recordings of excitatory postsynaptic potentials (e.p.s.p.'s) in a neuron, showing summation of successive e.p.s.p.'s. Each set of traces shows three superimposed responses. The arrow indicates the electrical stimulus used to trigger action potentials in the presynaptic neurons that make excitatory synapses onto the recorded cell. Trace a in each set shows a stimulus that failed to trigger the presynaptic input. Trace b shows e.p.s.p.'s that failed to reach threshold. Trace c shows summated e.p.s.p.'s that reach threshold and produce a postsynaptic action potential. In this figure, the postsynaptic cell is a motor neuron of the sympathetic nervous system (which is described in Chapter 11). (Unpublished data kindly provided by H.-S. Wang and D. McKinnon of the State University of New York at Stony Brook.)

cells produces only a small postsynaptic depolarization (Figure 8-4B). If several presynaptic cells fire simultaneously, however, their postsynaptic effects add up and can reach threshold. This type of summation is termed **spatial summation** to indicate that it occurs among spatially distinct inputs onto a single postsynaptic cell.

In the patellar reflex, both temporal and spatial summation are important in eliciting the reflexive response. In order to produce reflexive contraction of the quadriceps muscle, a tap to the patellar tendon must stretch the muscle sufficiently to fire a number of action potentials in each of a number of individual sensory neurons.

Some Possible Excitatory Neurotransmitters

The chemical neurotransmitter at the neuromuscular junction has been conclusively demonstrated to be acetylcholine, as discussed in the previous chapter. Acetylcholine is also used as a neurotransmitter at some neuron-to-neuron synapses, as well as at the neuromuscular junction. In addition, many other substances are excitatory neurotransmitters in the nervous system. The structures of some of the possible excitatory neurotransmitters are shown in Figure 8-5. Many of these neurotransmitters are relatively small molecules, often derived by simple chemical modifications to amino acids. Amino acids are more commonly thought of as the basic building blocks for the construction of proteins in the cell, but in the nervous system, amino acids are also often used for

(A)

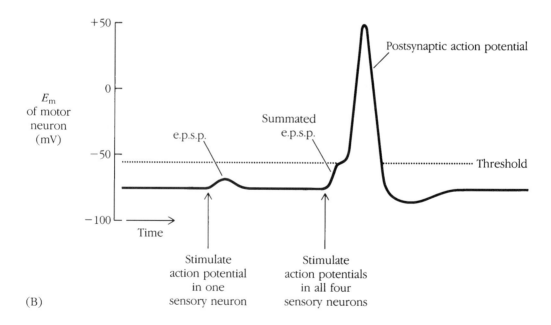

(B)

Figure 8-4

Spatial summation of excitatory inputs to a motor neuron. (A) Diagram of the synaptic circuitry and recording arrangement. (B) Illustration of synaptic responses in the postsynaptic motor neuron.

cell-to-cell signaling in neurotransmission. For example, glutamate and aspartate are unmodified amino acids, while norepinephrine and dopamine are derived from the amino acid tyrosine and serotonin is derived from tryptamine. There is evidence that glutamate may be the excitatory transmitter at the synapse be-

Glutamic acid
(Glutamate)

Acetylcholine

Norepinephrine

Aspartic acid
(Aspartate)

Serotonin
(5-hydroxytryptamine)

Dopamine

Arg-Pro-Lys-Pro-Gln-Gln-Phe-Phe-Gly-Leu-Met-NH$_2$

Substance P
(a string of 11 amino acids attached by peptide bonds)

Figure 8-5
Structures of some substances likely to be excitatory neurotransmitters in the nervous system.

tween the sensory and motor neurons in the patellar reflex. Other neurotransmitters are more structurally complex than the small amino acid derivatives and instead are formed from a whole series of individual amino acids linked by peptide bonds, like a small piece of a protein molecule. A representative member of this class is substance P, whose amino acid sequence is shown in Figure 8-5. Neurotransmitters of this type are called peptide neurotransmitters, or more simply **neuropeptides**. The list of excitatory neurotransmitters in Figure 8-5 is by no means exhaustive, and as information about the brain improves, it is likely that many new candidates will be added to the list.

Conductance-Decrease Excitatory Postsynaptic Potentials

In most cases, the mechanism by which an excitatory neurotransmitter produces an e.p.s.p. in the postsynaptic cell is the same as that by which acetylcholine depolarizes the muscle at the neuromuscular junction. That is, the transmitter opens channels in the postsynaptic membrane that allow sodium or sodium and potassium ions to cross. This alters the balance of sodium and potassium permeability so that the membrane potential shifts in a positive direction. In terms of the ionic current flowing across the postsynaptic membrane, the excitatory neurotransmitter acts to increase the relative sodium conductance of the postsynaptic membrane, so that the balance between inward sodium current and outward potassium current is struck slightly nearer E_{Na}. We learned in Chapter 4, however, that the membrane potential is controlled by the ratio of sodium to potassium permeability; thus, a depolarization might result either from an increase in sodium permeability or from a decrease in potassium permeability. Indeed, at some synapses, the effect of the transmitter is mediated via a reduction in the potassium conductance of the postsynaptic neuron. For instance, acetylcholine produces a long-lasting depolarization of sympathetic ganglion neurons in the frog. This depolarization is caused by a decrease in the potassium permeability of the neuron; acetylcholine closes a type of potassium channel in the neuron membrane, so that the outward potassium current across the membrane declines and the resting inward sodium current has a greater influence on membrane potential.

Inhibitory Synaptic Transmission

The Sensory Neuron to Antagonist Motor Neuron Synapse in the Patellar Reflex

The diagram for the patellar reflex that we have been considering since Chapter 5 is not really quite complete. As shown in Fig-

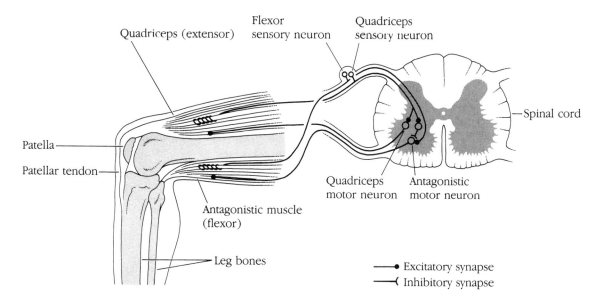

Figure 8-6
A revised diagram of the circuitry involved in stretch reflexes of thigh muscles.

ure 8-6, muscles other than the quadriceps must be taken into account for a more complete description. There are muscles at the back of the thigh that are attached to the lower leg bones and are responsible for flexion of the knee joint, just as the quadriceps is responsible for extension of the knee joint. These muscles are antagonistic to the action of the quadriceps. The antagonistic muscles have their own stretch-sensitive sensory neurons and motor neurons that are connected in a reflex chain just like those of the quadriceps. That is, a stretch of the muscle stimulates action potentials in the sensory neurons, which make excitatory synapses on the motor neurons that cause contraction of the same muscle.

As we've seen previously, when the patellar tendon is tapped, the quadriceps muscle reflexively contracts, causing the knee joint to extend (the "jerk" of the knee-jerk reflex). The extension of the joint stretches the flexor muscles at the back of the thigh, which should then contract because of the action of their own stretch reflex mechanism. The resulting flexion of the joint should stretch the quadriceps again and elicit reflexive extension, which should again elicit reflexive flexion, and so on. One might expect, then, that a single tap to the patellar tendon would send the knee joint into a series of oscillations that would continue until muscle exhaustion set in.

Why, then, does tapping the patellar tendon elicit only a single knee jerk? The answer lies in the more elaborate neuronal cir-

Figure 8-7

Inhibitory synaptic transmission between two neurons in the circuit of Figure 8-6. An action potential in the presynaptic neuron releases a neurotransmitter that hyperpolarizes the postsynaptic neuron. (A) Diagram of the synaptic circuitry and recording arrangement. (B) Postsynaptic response of the motor neuron.

(A)

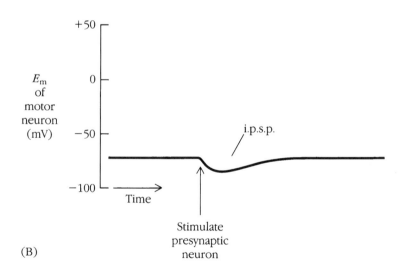

(B)

cuitry diagrammed in Figure 8-6. The nerve fibers of the stretch-sensitive sensory neurons from the quadriceps muscle actually branch profusely when they enter the spinal cord and make synaptic connections with many kinds of neurons in addition to the quadriceps motor neuron. Among these other synaptic connections is an excitatory synapse onto a type of neuron that makes an inhibitory synapse on the motor neurons of the antagonistic muscles. Thus, action potentials in quadriceps sensory neurons not only tend to excite quadriceps motor neurons but also tend indirectly to prevent antagonistic motor neurons from being excited by the antagonistic sensory neurons.

Characteristics of Inhibitory Synaptic Transmission

We now consider some of the properties of postsynaptic responses at an inhibitory synapse and then discuss the underlying mechanisms in the postsynaptic membrane. Figure 8-7 shows schematically an experimental arrangement to examine the inhibition of the antagonistic motor neuron in the patellar reflex. The membrane potential of the motor neuron is monitored with an intracellular probe while the inhibitory presynaptic neuron is stimulated electrically to fire action potentials. Presynaptically, the basic scheme for the release of the neurotransmitter is the same as that at other chemical synapses: The depolarization produced by the action potential allows calcium ions to enter the synaptic terminal through voltage-sensitive calcium channels, inducing synaptic vesicles containing the transmitter to fuse with the membrane of the terminal and release their contents. Postsynaptically, however, the effect of the transmitter is very different from that of acetylcholine at the neuromuscular junction. A sample result is shown in Figure 8-7B. An action potential in the presynaptic cell is followed by a transient increase in the postsynaptic membrane potential. When the membrane potential becomes more negative, the cell is said to be **hyperpolarized**. Because a hyperpolarization moves the membrane potential away from the threshold for firing an action potential, it is less likely that an excitatory input will be able to trigger an action potential, and the postsynaptic cell is inhibited. The change in membrane potential of the postsynaptic cell induced by the release of an inhibitory neurotransmitter is called an **inhibitory postsynaptic potential (i.p.s.p.)**.

Mechanism of Inhibition in the Postsynaptic Membrane

A recurring theme in the functioning of cells has been that changes in membrane potential are brought about by changes in ionic permeability of the plasma membrane. The i.p.s.p. is no different in this regard. *When the permeability of the membrane to a particular ion increases, the membrane potential tends to move toward the equilibrium potential for that ion.* We have already learned in

Figure 8-8
Mechanism by which an inhibitory postsynaptic potential might be produced in a postsynaptic neuron. (A) An increase in potassium permeability would be expected to cause a more negative membrane potential. (B) A neurotransmitter-activated potassium channel in the plasma membrane of a postsynaptic neuron at an inhibitory synapse.

(A)

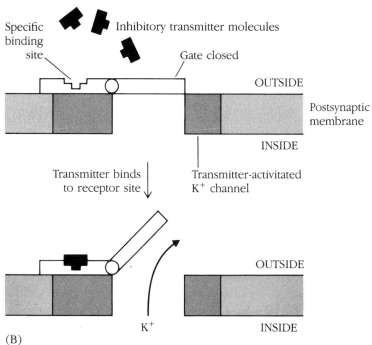

(B)

Chapter 5 how this sort of mechanism can explain the sequence of potential changes during an action potential. To see how a hyperpolarizing response might result from a change in ionic permeability, consider the situation diagrammed in Figure 8-8.

If potassium permeability of a cell membrane were suddenly increased, the membrane potential would be expected to move toward E_K, which is about -85 mV for a typical mammalian cell (see discussion in Chapters 3 and 4). In this situation, p_{Na}/p_K would be smaller than usual, and the balance between potassium and sodium would be closer to E_K. This is similar to the situation during the undershoot at the end of an action potential, when p_{Na}/p_K is transiently smaller than normal. As shown in Figure 8-8B, then, an inhibitory transmitter could hyperpolarize the postsynaptic cell by opening potassium channels in the postsynaptic membrane. As with acetylcholine at the neuromuscular junction, the inhibitory transmitter might act by combining with specific binding sites associated with the gate on the channel. When the binding sites are occupied, the gate controlling movement through the channel opens, and potassium ions can move out of the cell to drive E_m closer to the potassium equilibrium potential.

At most inhibitory synapses, however, it turns out that the transmitter-activated postsynaptic channels are not potassium channels. Instead, most inhibitory neurotransmitters open postsynaptic channels that allow chloride ions to cross the membrane. Recall from Chapters 3 and 4 that chloride pumps in the plasma membrane maintain the chloride equilibrium potential, E_{Cl}, at a more negative value than the resting membrane potential in many nerve cells. That is, the electrical gradient driving chloride out of the cell at the normal resting E_m is weaker than the concentration gradient driving chloride into the cell. Thus, if chloride channels open in the postsynaptic membrane, chloride ions will enter the cell, bringing negative charge into the cell and hyperpolarizing the neuron. An i.p.s.p. can result, then, from an increase in the chloride permeability of the postsynaptic cell.

In general terms, inhibition results when a neurotransmitter induces a permeability increase to an ion with an equilibrium potential that is more negative than the threshold level of membrane potential. This is because ions always move across the membrane in such a direction as to move E_m toward the equilibrium potential for that ion. If that equilibrium potential is more negative than the threshold, the ion will always *oppose* any attempt to reach threshold as soon as the depolarization exceeds the ion's equilibrium potential. Seen in this light, then, it is possible that an inhibitory

GABA
(γ-aminobutyric acid)

Glycine

Serotonin
(5-hydroxytryptamine)

Acetylcholine

Norepinephrine

Dopamine

Tyr-Gly-Gly-Phe-Leu
Leucine enkephalin
(a series of five amino acids connected by peptide bonds)

Figure 8-9
Structures of some substances likely to be inhibitory neurotransmitters in the nervous system.

permeability increase could occur without any visible change in membrane potential from the resting level. This could occur, for example, when the chloride equilibrium potential is equal to the resting potential. The effect of the inhibition would be revealed, however, if an excitatory input were activated while the inhibitory permeability increase is still active: The excitatory effect on membrane potential would be lessened because of the enhanced ability of chloride ions to oppose depolarization.

Some Possible Inhibitory Neurotransmitters

The identity of the chemical neurotransmitter at many inhibitory synapses within the nervous system remains unknown. However, several substances are likely candidates, and the structures of some of these are shown in Figure 8-9. Of those shown, γ-aminobutyric acid (GABA) and glycine are almost certainly transmitters at certain inhibitory synapses in the nervous system. Note that some of the candidates in Figure 8-9 also appeared in the list of candidate excitatory neurotransmitters in Figure 8-5. This is because a transmitter may have an excitatory effect on one type of neuron but an inhibitory effect on another type of neuron. Whether a substance is excitatory or inhibitory on a given neuron depends on the type of ion channel it opens in the postsynaptic membrane. If the transmitter-activated channel is a sodium or a sodium-potassium channel (as at the neuromuscular junction), the effect will be a depolarization and excitation; if the channel is a chloride or potassium channel, the effect will be hyperpolarization and inhibition. It is even possible for the same neurotransmitter to have opposite effects at two different synapses on the same postsynaptic neuron.

The Family of Neurotransmitter-Gated Ion Channels

In Chapter 7, we discussed the molecular structure of the acetylcholine-gated channel at the neuromuscular junction, and we saw that the channel is formed by the aggregation of several protein subunits. The other kinds of ion channels we have been describing here—those that underlie excitatory and inhibitory postsynaptic potentials—have also been studied at the molecular level, and like the acetylcholine-gated channel, these ion channels are formed by aggregates of individual subunits. Each type of subunit is coded by a specific gene. Nevertheless, the amino acid sequences of subunits making up the neurotransmitter-gated channels are more or less similar. For example, GABA-activated channels turn out to be structurally similar to glycine-activated channels and to acetylcholine-activated channels; glutamate-activated channels also are related to acetylcholine-activated channels, although more distantly. The genes coding for the subunits of the ion channels opened by neurotransmitters form a related family of genes, which is called the **ligand-gated ion channel**

family to indicate that members of the family form ion channels that are opened by the binding of a chemical signal (the ligand) to a specific binding site on the channel.

Of course, there are also important functional differences among the members of this gene family. First, there must be specificity for activation by a particular neurotransmitter: A glutamate-activated channel is not activated by GABA, even though a comparison of Figures 8-5 and 8-9 shows that glutamate and GABA are structurally quite similar. (Indeed, GABA is formed enzymatically by modification of glutamate.) Thus, there must be unique features of the part of the protein that forms the binding site for each type of neurotransmitter-gated channel. Second, there must be important differences among members of the ligand-gated ion channel family in the properties of the pore through which ions can cross the membrane when the channel is open. Some ligand-gated channels form cation pores (e.g., glutamate channels or acetylcholine channels), while others form anion pores (e.g., glycine or GABA channels). This difference in ionic selectivity must reflect underlying differences in how the pore region is constructed.

Indirect Actions of Neurotransmitters

In all of our discussions of neurotransmitter action, both at the neuromuscular junction (see Chapter 7) and in the central nervous system (in this chapter), we have considered only direct effects of the transmitter on the ionic permeability of the postsynaptic cell. In such direct actions, the receptor (binding site) to which the neurotransmitter molecules bind is part of the ion channel protein itself (see Figures 7-4 and 8-8). However, there is a wide variety of postsynaptic effects of neurotransmitters in which the receptor is a separate protein from the ion channel and the linkage between the two is indirect. Such mechanisms allow a single neurotransmitter to have various and diverse effects on a postsynaptic neuron, such as closing one type of ion channel while opening another type, affecting the metabolism of the postsynaptic cell as well as its membrane permeability, altering gene expression, and so on. The basic scheme for such indirect actions is shown in Figure 8-10. The first two steps (presynaptic release of neurotransmitter and binding of neurotransmitter to specific postsynaptic receptor) are no different from the direct actions of neurotransmitter that we considered earlier. What happens next, however, is quite different; the combination of the transmitter with its receptor causes the postsynaptic cell

1. Neurotransmitter is released by presynaptic neuron

2. Neurotransmitter combines with specific receptor in membrane of postsynaptic neuron

3. Combination of neurotransmitter with receptor leads to intracellular release or production of a second messenger

4. Second messenger interacts (directly or indirectly) with ion channel, causing it to open or close

Figure 8-10
Overview of the indirect linkage of a neurotransmitter to activity of an ion channel via an intracellular second messenger in the postsynaptic cell.

to release internally a substance, called a second messenger (the neurotransmitter being the first messenger), that alters the state of the postsynaptic cell. There is an ever-growing list of second messenger molecules, as we learn more about the basic cell biology of indirect neurotransmitter actions. These include cyclic adenosine monophosphate (cyclic AMP), which is produced from ATP by the enzyme adenylate cyclase; cyclic guanosine monophosphate (cyclic GMP), which is produced from the guanine nucleotide equivalent of ATP (GTP) by the enzyme guanylate cyclase; the dual second messengers diacylglycerol and inositol trisphosphate, both of which are produced from a particular kind of membrane lipid molecule by the enzyme phospholipase C; and arachidonic acid, which is produced from membrane lipid by the enzyme phospholipase A.

The effect that the second messenger then has on the cell depends on the specific case under consideration. If the second messenger causes opening of a sodium channel or closing of a potassium channel, for instance, the postsynaptic neuron would tend to be excited; conversely, if the second messenger leads to opening of a potassium or chloride channel, or to closing of a sodium channel, then the net result would be inhibition of the postsynaptic cell. What is the linkage between the second messenger and the target ion channel? In some instances, the second messenger itself directly combines with the ion channel, causing it to open. This happens in the photoreceptor cells of the retina, where cyclic GMP opens a type of sodium channel in the plasma membrane. In other instances, the second messenger acts indirectly, by activating an enzyme that in turn affects the ion channel. This is usually the case, for example, with cyclic AMP, which activates an enzyme called cyclic AMP–dependent protein kinase (or protein kinase A); the protein kinase phosphorylates proteins, including ion channels, which is a common biochemical mechanism by which protein function is altered. (Phosphorylation means that inorganic phosphate, derived from splitting ATP into ADP + phosphate, is attached to a specific site on the target protein by the protein kinase enzyme.) In neurons, for example, phosphorylation of voltage-activated calcium channels is thought to be necessary for normal operation of the channel (that is, phosphorylated channels are able to open upon depolarization, while nonphosphorylated channels are inactive); thus, a neurotransmitter might indirectly affect calcium channel function in a postsynaptic cell by altering the level of cyclic AMP.

We have seen that binding of a neurotransmitter to its postsynaptic receptor can lead to activation of an enzyme that produces a second messenger, which in turn can directly or indirectly affect ion permeability of the postsynaptic cell. What is the nature of the linkage between the activated receptor and the enzyme that makes the second messenger? Here, again, the linkage is indirect. There is yet another membrane protein involved, called a GTP binding protein (or G-protein, for short) because binding of GTP is required for the G-protein to be activated. In its inactivated state, the G-protein has GDP bound to it; the activated neurotransmitter receptor catalyzes the replacement of GDP by GTP and thus the activation of the G-protein. The activated G-protein then interacts with and stimulates the enzyme producing the second messenger (adenylate cyclase in the case of cyclic AMP, for example). There are various kinds of G-proteins, each with specific effects on specific target enzymes; some G-proteins stimulate the activity of the target enzyme, while others inhibit it. Thus, neurotransmitter activation of one receptor might increase the level of a second messenger, while activation of a different receptor might decrease the level of the second messenger, depending on the type of G-protein to which the receptor is coupled. In addition to acting via second messengers, there is also evidence that activated G-protein may itself in some cases be a messenger that directly activates ion channels.

All of these indirect actions of neurotransmitters are summarized by the sequence of events shown in Figure 8-11. We can think of this sequence as an enzymatic cascade, where an activated neurotransmitter receptor acts as an enzyme to activate G-protein, which in turn activates an enzyme that produces a second messenger, which in turn activates another enzyme that affects ion channel operation. In this sequence, there are three

1. Neurotransmitter is released by presynaptic neuron

2. Neurotransmitter combines with specific receptor in membrane of postsynaptic neuron

3. Activated receptor activates G-protein

4A. Activated G-protein acts on enzyme that produces second messenger (e.g., adenylate cyclase)

4B. Activated G-protein directly combines with and activates ion channel

5. Level of second messenger increases (excitatory G-protein) or decreases (inhibitory G-protein) in postsynaptic cell

6A. Second messenger activates an enzyme (e.g., protein kinase A)

6B. Second messenger directly acts on ion channel

7. Activated enzyme acts on ion channel to alter its function (opens channel, closes channel, or makes channel capable of responding to a stimulus, such as depolarization)

Figure 8-11
The sequence of events in the indirect action of a neurotransmitter on membrane permeability of a postsynaptic cell. Ion channel activity may be altered by G-proteins, by second messengers, or by second messenger–dependent enzymes.

points at which an effect on an ion channel might be found. First, activated G-protein might bind to and activate an ion channel. Second, the second messenger might directly bind to the channel. Third, an enzyme, such as a protein kinase, that depends on the presence of the second messenger might act on the ion channel. In all cases, the net excitatory or inhibitory effect of the neurotransmitter in question will depend on what kind of ion channel is affected in the postsynaptic membrane and on whether the ion channel tends to be activated or inactivated by the indirect action of the neurotransmitter.

Presynaptic Inhibition and Facilitation

A different type of inhibitory interaction is sometimes observed among neurons in the nervous system. In the inhibition we discussed earlier (see Figure 8-8), the inhibition is accomplished by altering directly the membrane permeability of the postsynaptic cell. In the other type of inhibition, the inhibition is exerted indirectly by affecting the membrane of an excitatory presynaptic terminal. This type of inhibition is called **presynaptic inhibition**, and is illustrated schematically in Figure 8-12. In this situation, the inhibitory terminal acts to reduce the influx of calcium into the excitatory synaptic terminal during an action potential. This in turn causes fewer synaptic vesicles to fuse with the membrane of the excitatory terminal and thus reduces the release of excitatory transmitter onto the postsynaptic neuron. The reduction of calcium influx into the excitatory terminal can be caused by the inhibitory input in a number of ways. One possible mechanism is to reduce the depolarization produced by an action potential in the excitatory presynaptic terminal. A smaller depolarization opens fewer voltage-sensitive calcium channels, so that less calcium enters the excitatory terminal. Another possibility would be to decrease the number of voltage-sensitive calcium channels that are in the phosphorylated state (see previous section) and are thus capable of opening upon depolarization. It would also be possible to reduce the calcium influx by decreasing the duration of the action potential in the presynaptic terminal; this might be done, for instance, by increasing the number of voltage-sensitive potassium channels, thus giving more rapid repolarization during the action potential. The electron micrograph of Figure 8-12B shows a synapse on a nerve fiber at a location where that fiber in turn makes a synapse onto another postsynaptic neuron. This kind of arrangement might underlie the presynaptic inhibition of the type just described.

Of course, a synapse onto a synapse like the arrangement shown in Figure 8-12 might also be used to facilitate the release of neurotransmitter from the excitatory terminal. This **presynaptic facilitation** is known to occur, for example, in the nervous system of a sea slug, *Aplysia*, where the neurotransmitter serotonin increases the effectiveness of an excitatory synaptic connection from a presynaptic sensory neuron onto a postsynaptic motor neuron. Serotonin does this by inhibiting (indirectly via a second messenger) a type of voltage-sensitive potassium channel in the presynaptic neuron. When the potassium channel is inhibited, the repolarizing phase of the presynaptic action potential is slowed, giving a prolonged depolarization and thus greater presynaptic calcium influx and enhanced transmitter release.

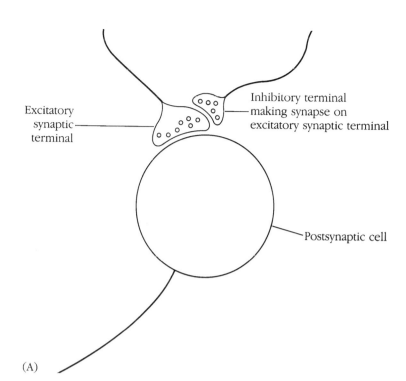

Excitatory synaptic terminal

Inhibitory terminal making synapse on excitatory synaptic terminal

Postsynaptic cell

(A)

Figure 8-12
(A) Schematic arrangement for presynaptic inhibition in the nervous system. The inhibitory terminal makes synaptic contact with another synaptic terminal, rather than directly with the postsynaptic cell. (B) Electron micrograph showing a synapse (Terminal 1) in the vertebrate central nervous system onto an axon (Terminal 2) that in turn makes a synapse onto a third neuronal process (labeled "d" for dendrite). The arrows show the direction of synaptic transmission from terminal 1 to terminal 2 and from terminal 2 to the dendrite. Note the accumulations of synaptic vesicles in terminals 1 and 2. (Part B reproduced with permission from Wickelgren WO. Physiological and anatomical characteristics of reticulospinal neurones in lamprey. *J. Physiol* 1977;270 89–114.)

(B) 0.5 μm

(A)

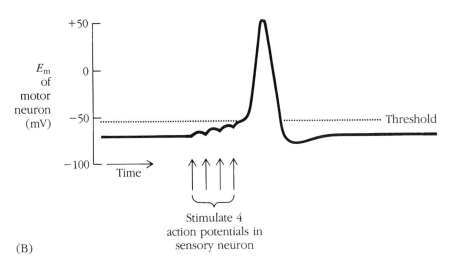

(B)

Figure 8-13

Integration of excitatory and inhibitory synaptic inputs by a neuron in the nervous system. (A) Experimental arrangement for the measurements shown in (B), (C), and (D). (B) Stimulating the excitatory presynaptic neuron produces a postsynaptic action potential if there is sufficient temporal summation to reach threshold. (C) Stimulating the inhibitory presynaptic neuron prevents the excitatory inputs in (B) from reaching threshold. (D) The inhibitory effect can be overcome by increasing the amount of excitatory stimulation.

(C)

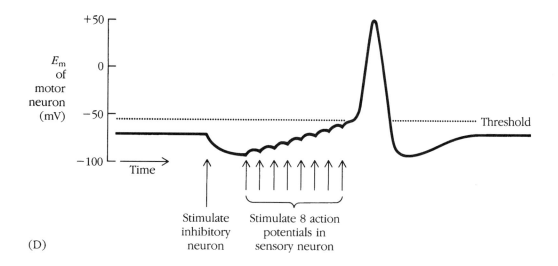

(D)

Neuronal Integration

In the nervous system, neurons receive both excitatory and inhibitory synaptic inputs. The decision of a postsynaptic neuron to fire an action potential is determined by only one factor: whether or not the threshold level of membrane potential has been reached. This is determined at any instant by the sum of all existing excitatory and inhibitory synaptic potentials. This can be seen by looking once again at the antagonistic motor neuron in the patellar reflex, as shown in Figure 8-13.

When the sensory neuron from the antagonistic muscle is stimulated to fire action potentials, e.p.s.p.'s result in the motor neuron that controls the antagonist muscle, and an action potential will occur if there is sufficient temporal summation among the e.p.s.p.'s. If the inhibitory neuron is stimulated at the same time, however, the same series of excitatory inputs might not be able to reach threshold. This inhibitory effect could be overcome by increasing the strength of the excitatory input, either by increasing the number of presynaptic action potentials in the sensory neuron or by increasing the number of sensory neurons activated. It is the balance between the excitatory and inhibitory inputs that governs whether or not a postsynaptic action potential is generated.

The process of summing, or integrating, all the synaptic inputs onto a neuron is called **neuronal integration**, and it underlies all the information transfer and processing capabilities of the nervous system. The information processing capacity of a single neuron is considerable in that a typical neuron receives hundreds or thousands of synapses from hundreds or thousands of other neurons and makes synaptic connections itself with an equal number of postsynaptic neurons. This capacity is increased still further by the fact that synaptic inputs to a cell have widely varying weights: Some synapses produce large changes in postsynaptic membrane potential, while others cause only tiny changes. Further, the weight given a particular input might vary with time, as in the case of presynaptic inhibition. A network of some 10^{10} of these sophisticated units, like the human brain, has staggering information processing ability.

Summary

Chemical synapses between neurons in the nervous system are similar to the synapse at the neuromuscular junction in the following ways:

1. Neurotransmitter is stored in the synaptic terminal in membrane-bound synaptic vesicles.
2. Influx of external calcium ions into the terminal is a necessary step in the release of neurotransmitter.
3. Fusion of the synaptic vesicle with the plasma membrane of the terminal is the mechanism of transmitter release.
4. Neurotransmitter molecules combine with specific postsynaptic receptors and open ion channels in the postsynaptic membrane.

Nervous system synapses are different from the neuromuscular junction in the following ways:

1. At most synapses, a single presynaptic action potential produces only a small change in postsynaptic membrane potential. At the neuromuscular junction, a single presynaptic action potential produces a large depolarization of the muscle cell and triggers a postsynaptic action potential.

2. Synapses between neurons can be either excitatory or inhibitory.

3. Acetylcholine is probably the neurotransmitter at a few synapses between neurons, but a host of other substances are also probably neurotransmitters in the nervous system.

4. A skeletal muscle cell receives synaptic input from only one neuron, a single motor neuron. A neuron in the nervous system may receive synaptic connections from thousands of different neurons. The output of a neuron depends on the integration of all the inhibitory and excitatory inputs active at a given instant.

5. At the neuromuscular junction, acetylcholine combines with postsynaptic binding sites that are part of the channel protein and directly opens the channel. In the central nervous system, a neurotransmitter may have either a direct effect on an ion channel or an indirect effect via an internal second messenger in the postsynaptic cell.

CELLULAR PHYSIOLOGY OF MUSCLE CELLS

This section is concerned with the second major type of excitable cell: muscle cells. These cells are specialized to produce movement when they are electrically stimulated, and their actions are the most obvious external manifestation of the activities of the nervous system. The point of interaction between the nervous and muscular systems—the neuromuscular junction—was the central focus for the discussion of chemical synaptic transmission in Chapter 7. In the first chapter of Part III, Chapter 9, we return to the neuromuscular junction to examine the sequence of events that link an action potential in the postsynaptic muscle cell to mechanical contraction. This linkage is the process called **excitation-contraction coupling**, and the explanation of this process in terms of underlying molecular mechanisms stands as one of the major accomplishments of modern cellular physiology. In Chapter 10 we discuss some of the characteristics of contractions of whole skeletal muscles and how the strength of contraction is controlled by the nervous system. Chapter 11 considers some of the important electrical differences between the cells of skeletal muscles and the muscle cells of the heart. These electrical differences underlie the ability of the heart as an organ to produce the rhythmic, coordinated contractions necessary to pump the blood through the body. The control of the heart by the autonomic nervous system is also considered in Chapter 11.

9

Excitation–Contraction Coupling in Skeletal Muscle

Throughout Part II of the book, we used the patellar reflex as an example system to explore the cellular signals underlying nervous system function. The final stage of the patellar reflex is the contraction of the quadriceps muscle brought about by the activity of the motor neurons making excitatory synaptic connections with that muscle. The arrival of an action potential in the synaptic terminal of the presynaptic motor neuron causes release of the chemical neurotransmitter acetylcholine. Acetylcholine in turn depolarizes the end-plate region of the postsynaptic muscle cell, initiating an action potential in the muscle cell. This action potential propagates along the long, thin muscle cell just as the neuron action potential propagates along nerve fibers. The muscle action potential serves as the trigger for the contraction of the muscle cell. This chapter examines the events that intervene between the occurrence of the action potential in the plasma membrane of the muscle cell and the activation of the contraction: the process of excitation–contraction coupling. Then, in Chapter 10 we look at how the motor nervous system is organized to integrate the twitch-like contractions of individual muscle fibers into the smooth and graded contractions of a muscle as a whole.

To begin, it is useful to examine the structure of the muscle cells at the level of both the light and the electron microscope. We then consider the molecular make-up of the contractile apparatus and discuss the biochemical mechanisms that control the action of that apparatus. The chapter concludes with a discussion of how the action potential of the muscle cell is coupled to the contractile machinery to produce the muscle contraction.

Figure 9-1
Microscopic structure of skeletal muscle. Muscle components are viewed at increasing magnification in (A) through (D).

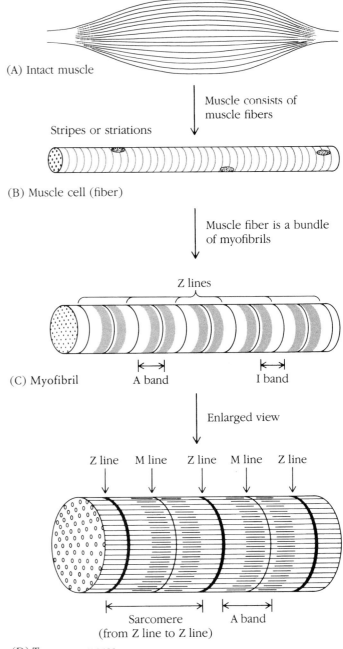

(A) Intact muscle

Muscle consists of muscle fibers

Stripes or striations

(B) Muscle cell (fiber)

Muscle fiber is a bundle of myofibrils

Z lines

(C) Myofibril   A band   I band

Enlarged view

Z line   M line   Z line   M line   Z line

Sarcomere   A band
(from Z line to Z line)

(D) Two sarcomeres

The Three Types of Muscle

There are two general classes of muscle in the body: striated and smooth. Both are named for the characteristic appearance of the individual cells making up the muscle tissue when viewed through a microscope; striated muscle cells (Figure 9-1) have closely spaced, crosswise stripes (striations), but smooth muscle cells do not and thus appear smooth. Smooth muscle is found in the gut, blood vessels, the uterus, and other locations in which contractions are usually slow and maintained. The muscles that move and support the skeletal framework of the body—the skeletal muscles—are made up of striated muscle cells. This chapter focuses on the structure and properties of skeletal muscle cells.

The cells that make up the muscle of the heart are also striated, like skeletal muscle. Because the membranes of cardiac muscle cells are electrically quite different from those of skeletal muscle cells, cardiac muscle is usually regarded as a distinct class of muscle in its own right. The characteristics of cardiac muscle are discussed in Chapter 11.

Structure of Skeletal Muscle

Figure 9-1 shows the structure of a typical mammalian skeletal muscle at progressively greater magnification. To the naked eye, an intact muscle appears to be vaguely striped longitudinally, as in Figure 9-1A. Upon closer inspection, the muscle is made up of bundles of individual cells: the muscle cells or muscle fibers (see Figure 9-1B). In mammalian muscle, the individual cells are about 50 µm in diameter and are typically as long as the whole muscle. Thus, muscle cells are long, thin fibers. Because the end-plate region extends over only a few micrometers, a rapidly propagating action potential, like that of a nerve cell, is required in skeletal muscle cells to pass along the motor neuron's command to contract.

Individual muscle cells consist of bundles of still smaller fibers called myofibrils. Thus, the plasma membrane of a single muscle cell encloses many myofibrils. At the level of the myofibrils, the structural basis of the crosswise striations of skeletal muscle cells begins to become apparent. As shown in Figure 9-1C, myofibrils exhibit a repeating pattern of crosswise light and dark stripes. Early anatomists who first described these stripes had no idea of their function and gave them the names A band, I band, and Z line. The I band is a predominantly light region with the dark Z line at its center, while the A band is a darker region separating two I bands of the repeating pattern. At still higher magnification, the A band can be seen to have its own internal structure (see Figure 9-1D); two darker areas at the outer edges of the A band are separated by a lighter region with a faint dark line, called the M line, at the center. The basic unit of the repeating striation pattern of a myofibril is called a sarcomere, and it is defined as extending from one Z line to the next—that is, from the center of one I band to the center of the next I band. Thus, Figure 9-1D shows two complete sarcomeres along the length of a single myofibril.

Changes in Striation Pattern on Contraction

All of these myofibril striation patterns would be rather uninteresting, except to anatomists, if it weren't for the important observation that the relation among the stripes changes when a muscle cell contracts. This change can best be appreciated at the level of the electron microscope, as shown diagrammatically in Figure 9-2. Through the electron microscope, a myofibril can be seen to consist of two kinds of longitudinally oriented filaments, called thick and thin filaments. Both the thick and thin filaments are arrayed in parallel groups. As shown in Figure 9-2, the Z line corresponds to the position where the thin filaments of one sarcomere join onto those of the neighboring sarcomere and where cross-connections are made among the parallel thin filaments. The thick filaments within a sarcomere are joined to each other at the M line. It is clear from comparing Figure 9-2 with Figure 9-1D that the lighter I band corresponds to the region occupied only by thin filaments, and the darker A band corresponds to the spatial extent of the thick filaments. The darker regions at the two edges of the A band correspond to the region of overlap of the thick and thin filaments. The thick filaments bear thin fibers that appear to link to the thin filaments in the region of overlap, forming cross-bridges between the thick and thin filaments.

Upon contraction, the length of each sarcomere shortens—that is, the distance between successive Z lines diminishes. However, the width of the A band is unaffected by contraction; thus, only the I band becomes thinner during a contraction. In terms of the thick and thin filaments, this observation can be explained by the sliding filament hypothesis, which is illustrated in Figure 9-2B.

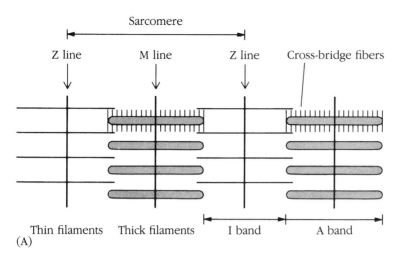

Sarcomere

Z line   M line   Z line   Cross-bridge fibers

Thin filaments   Thick filaments   I band   A band
(A)

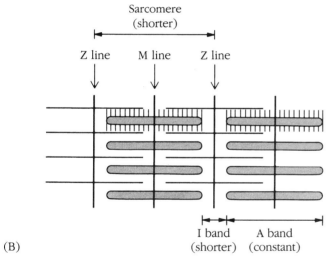

Sarcomere
(shorter)

Z line   M line   Z line

I band   A band
(shorter)   (constant)

(B)

Figure 9-2
Schematic representation of the relationships between thick and thin filaments of a myofibril in (A) a relaxed muscle and (B) a contracted muscle.

Neither the thick nor the thin filaments change in length during a contraction; rather, shortening occurs because the filaments slide with respect to one another, so that the region of overlap increases. In order to understand how the sliding occurs, it is necessary to examine the molecular make-up of the thick and thin filaments.

Molecular Composition of Filaments

The thick filaments are aggregates of a protein called myosin, which consists of a long fibrous "tail" connected to a globular

Figure 9-3

Diagram of the structure of a single molecule of the thick filament protein myosin. The fibrous tail is connected to the globular head region via a flexible connection point. The globular head includes a region that can bind and split a molecule of ATP.

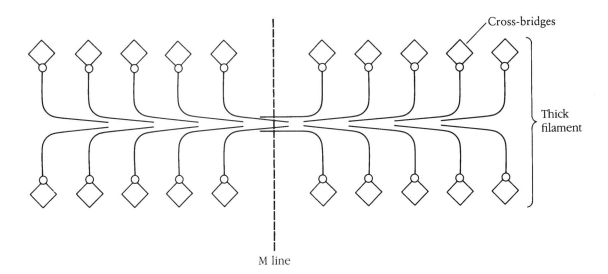

Figure 9-4

Hypothetical structure of a thick filament. The fibrous tails of individual myosin molecules polymerize to form the backbone of the filament. The globular heads radiate out perpendicularly to the long axis of the filament to form the cross-bridges to the thin filament. The myosin molecules reverse orientation at the M line.

"head" region, as shown schematically in Figure 9-3. The fibrous tails tend to aggregate into long filaments, with the heads projecting off to the side. Figure 9-4 shows a generally accepted view of how myosin molecules are arranged in the thick filaments of a sarcomere. The aggregated tails form the backbone of the thick filament, and the globular heads form the cross-bridges that connect with adjacent thin filaments.

The globular head of myosin contains a region that can bind adenosine triphosphate (ATP) and split one of the high-energy phosphate bonds of ATP, releasing the stored chemical energy. That is, myosin acts as an ATPase that hydrolyzes ATP to yield adenosine diphosphate (ADP) plus inorganic phosphate (P_i). The energy provided by ATP is transferred to the myosin molecule, which is transformed into an "energized" state. This sequence can be summarized as follows:

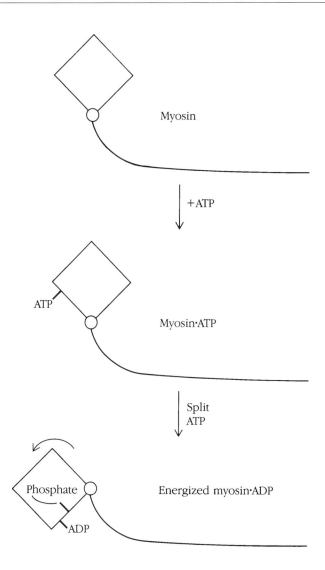

Figure 9-5
A molecule of myosin can bind a molecule of ATP. Energy released by splitting a high-energy phosphate bond of the ATP is used to form an energized form of myosin. The transition from a resting to an energized state involves rotation of the globular head about its flexible attachment site to the fibrous tail.

$$\text{Myosin} + \text{ATP} \rightarrow \text{Myosin·ATP} \rightarrow \text{Energized Myosin·ADP} + P_i$$

Here, the dot indicates that two molecules are bound together, as in an enzyme-substrate complex. To make a mechanical analogy, the globular head behaves as though it is attached to the fibrous tail at a hinged connection point. The energy released by ATP causes the head to pivot about the hinge into the energized state, as drawn schematically in Figure 9-5. To continue with mechanical analogies, this can be thought of as cocking the spring-loaded hammer of a cap pistol. As we will see shortly, the energy stored in this energized form of myosin is the energy that fuels the sliding of the filaments during contraction.

The thin filaments within a myofibril are largely made up of the protein actin. Thin filaments also contain two other kinds of protein molecules called troponin and tropomyosin, whose roles in contraction are discussed a bit later; for the present we concentrate on the actin molecules. Actin is a globular protein that polymerizes to form long chains; thus, the thin filament can be thought of as a long string of actin molecules, like a pearl necklace. (Actually, each thin filament consists of two actin chains entwined about each other in a helix, but for a conceptual understanding of the sliding filament hypothesis it is not necessary to keep this in mind.) Each actin molecule in the chain contains a binding site that can combine with a specific site on the globular head of a myosin molecule. This is the site of attachment of the cross-bridge on the thin filament.

Interaction Between Myosin and Actin

When actin combines with energized myosin, the stored energy in the myosin molecule is released. This causes the myosin molecule to return to its resting state, and the globular head pivots about its hinged attachment point to the thick filament. The pivoting motion requires that the thick and thin filaments move longitudinally with respect to each other. This mechanical analogue is illustrated schematically in Figure 9-6. The exact nature of the chemical changes in a myosin molecule during the transition from a resting to an energized state and back is unknown at present; the sliding filament hypothesis, however, requires that there be some chemical equivalent of the hinged arrangement shown in Figure 9-6.

How is the bond between actin and myosin broken so that a new cycle of sliding can be initiated? In the scheme presented so far, each myosin molecule on the thick filament could interact only one time with an actin molecule on the thin filament, and the total excursion of sliding would be restricted to that produced by a single pivoting of the globular head. In order to produce the large movements of the filaments that actually occur, it is necessary that the attachment of the cross-bridges be broken so that the cycle of myosin energization, binding to actin, and movement can be repeated. The full cycle that allows this to occur is summar-

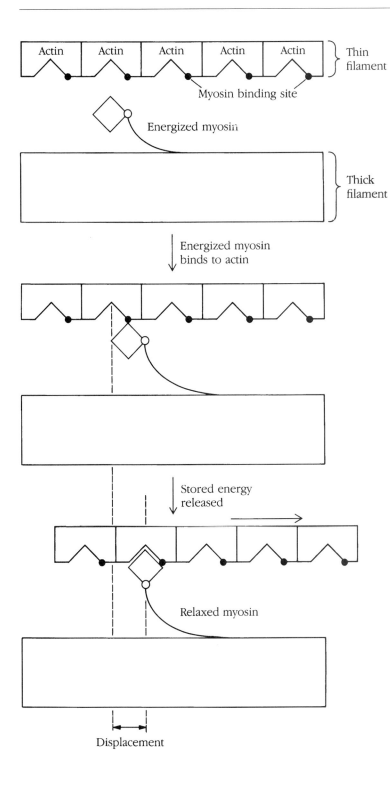

Figure 9-6
Schematic representation of the interaction between energized myosin and actin according to the sliding filament hypothesis. Energized myosin binds to a specific binding site on actin, and the stored energy is released. The resulting relaxation of the myosin molecule entails rotation about the flexible attachment site to the rest of the thick filament. The rotation induces longitudinal sliding of the filaments. The fibrous tail connecting the myosin molecule to the rest of the thick filament is assumed to be "springy," so that the globular head can reach across to the cross-bridge attachment site on the thin filament.

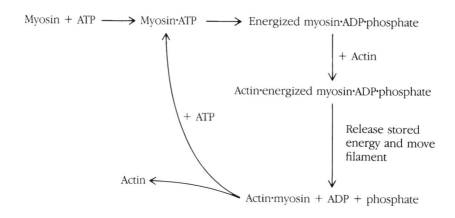

Figure 9-7
The cycle of cross-bridge formation and dissociation between myosin and actin during filament sliding.

ized in Figure 9-7. When energized myosin binds to actin and releases its stored energy, the ADP bound to the ATPase site of the globular head is released. This allows a new molecule of ATP to bind to the myosin. When this happens, the bond between actin and myosin is broken, possibly because of structural changes in the globular head induced by the interaction between ATP and myosin. The new ATP molecule can then be split by myosin to regenerate the energized form, which is then free to interact with another actin molecule on the chain making up the thin filament. Note that there are two roles for ATP in this scheme: to provide the energy to "cock" myosin for movement, and to break the interaction between actin and myosin after movement has occurred. If there is no ATP present, actin and myosin get stuck together and a rigid muscle results (as in rigor mortis).

Each of the many myosin heads on an individual thick filament independently goes through repetitive cycles of energization by ATP, binding to actin, releasing of stored energy to produce sliding, and detachment from actin. Each cycle results in the splitting of one molecule of ATP to ADP and inorganic phosphate. Note from Figure 9-4 that the orientation of the myosin heads reverses at the midpoint of the thick filament, the M line. This is the proper orientation to pull both Z lines at the boundary of a sarcomere toward the center (Figure 9-8). The thin filaments attached to the left Z line will be pulled to the right by the cyclical pivoting of the myosin cross-bridges. Similarly, the thin filaments attached to the right Z line will be pulled to the left. Thus, each sarcomere in each myofibril shortens, and the whole muscle shortens.

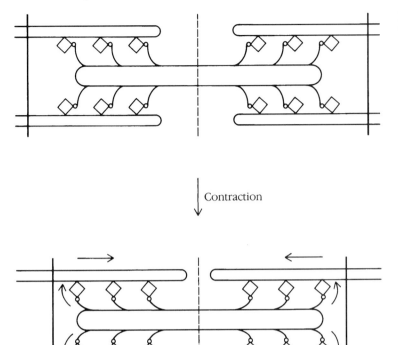

Contraction

Figure 9-8
The mechanism of sarcomere
shortening during contraction
according to the sliding filament
hypothesis. For clarity, the
myosin heads are shown acting
in concert, although in reality
they behave independently.

Regulation of Contraction

In the scheme summarized in Figure 9-7, there is no mechanism
to control the interaction between actin and myosin. That is, as
long as ATP is present, we would expect every muscle in the body
to be in a perpetual state of maximum contraction. This section
examines the molecular mechanisms that prevent the interaction
of actin with myosin except when a contraction is triggered by an
action potential in the muscle cell membrane.

Recall that thin filaments also contain the proteins troponin and
tropomyosin. These proteins are responsible for regulating the
interaction between individual myosin and actin molecules in the
thick and thin filaments. The regulatory scheme is summarized by
the diagrams in Figure 9-9. In the resting muscle, tropomyosin is
in a position on the thin filament that allows it to effectively cover
the myosin binding site on actin. Myosin's access to the binding
site is blocked by tropomyosin. The position of tropomyosin on

Figure 9-9
Regulation of the interaction between actin and myosin by calcium ions, troponin, and tropomyosin. In the absence of calcium ions, access to the myosin binding site of actin is prevented by tropomyosin. When calcium binds to troponin, the binding site is accessible and the sliding interaction is allowed.

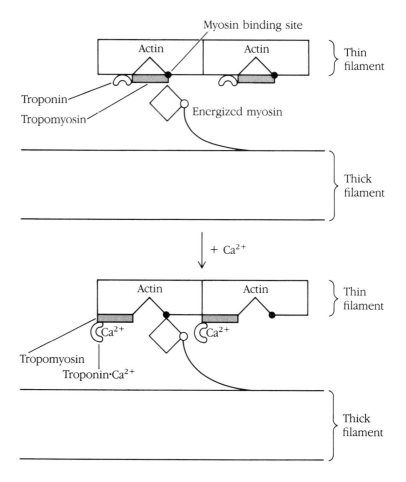

the actin polymer is in turn regulated by troponin. In the resting state, troponin locks tropomyosin in the blocking position. Thus, tropomyosin acts like a trapdoor covering the myosin binding site, and troponin acts like a lock to keep the door from opening.

What is the trigger that causes tropomyosin to reveal the myosin binding sites on actin? The signal that initiates contraction is the binding of calcium ions to troponin. Each troponin molecule contains a specific binding site for a single calcium ion. Normally, the concentration of calcium inside the cell is very low, and the binding site is not occupied. It is in this state that troponin locks tropomyosin in the blocking position. When an action potential occurs in the muscle cell plasma membrane, however, the concentration of calcium ions in the ICF rises dramatically, and calcium binds to troponin. When this happens, there is a structural change in the troponin molecule, and the interaction between troponin and tropomyosin is altered in such a way that tropomyosin uncovers the myosin binding site on actin. The cycle of events depicted in Figure 9-7 is then allowed to occur, and the filaments slide past each other.

The Sarcoplasmic Reticulum

Where does the calcium come from to trigger the interaction of actin and myosin underlying the sliding of the filaments? Recall from Chapter 7 that a rise in internal calcium is also responsible for the release of chemical transmitter molecules during synaptic transmission, and that in that case the calcium enters the cell from the ECF through voltage-sensitive calcium channels in the plasma membrane. In the case of skeletal muscle, however, the calcium does not come from outside the cell; rather, the calcium is injected into the ICF from a separate intracellular compartment called the sarcoplasmic reticulum. The sarcoplasmic reticulum is an intracellular sack that surrounds the myofibrils of a muscle cell. This sack forms a separate intracellular compartment, bounded by its own membrane that is not continuous with the plasma membrane of the muscle cell.

The concentration of calcium ions inside the sarcoplasmic reticulum is much higher than it is in the rest of the space inside the cell; in fact, it is probably higher than the concentration of calcium in the ECF. This accumulation of calcium inside the sarcoplasmic reticulum is accomplished by a calcium pump in the membrane of the sarcoplasmic reticulum. Like the sodium pump of the plasma membrane, this calcium pump uses metabolic energy in the form of ATP to transport calcium ions across the membrane against a large concentration gradient; in this case, the pump moves calcium ions into the sarcoplasmic reticulum. To initiate a contraction, a puff of calcium ions is released from the sarcoplasmic reticulum, which is strategically located surrounding the contractile apparatus of the myofibrils. The action of the released calcium is terminated as the ions are pumped back into the sarcoplasmic reticulum by the calcium pump. Here, then, is a third role for ATP in the contraction process: ATP, as the fuel for the calcium pump, is responsible for terminating a contraction as well as for energizing myosin and breaking the bond between actin and myosin.

Calcium is released from the sarcoplasmic reticulum via calcium-selective ion channels, which are located in the sarcoplasmic reticulum membrane. These calcium channels are quite different from the voltage-dependent calcium channels we encountered previously in our discussion of synaptic transmission. Rather than being activated by depolarization, as are the voltage-dependent calcium channels, these calcium channels in the sarcoplasmic reticulum are activated by an increase in cytoplasmic calcium concentration. For this reason, they are referred to as calcium-induced calcium release channels. If calcium is released from the sarcoplasmic reticulum via channels that are themselves activated by an increase in calcium, then the calcium release process exhibits positive feedback reminiscent of the rising phase of the action potential (where depolarization opens sodium channels, which in turn produce further depolarization). This ensures that the calcium release will rapidly rise, producing fast and complete activation of the contraction mechanism.

The Transverse Tubule System

How does an action potential in the plasma membrane of a muscle cell trigger release of calcium from the sarcoplasmic reticulum? It has been demonstrated that the crucial aspect of the action potential in triggering contraction is depolarization of the plasma membrane; any manipulation that produces depolarization can cause contraction. How can depolarization of the plasma membrane at the outer surface of the cell affect sarcoplasmic reticulum surrounding myofibrils deep in the interior of the muscle cell? The answer is that there are periodic infoldings, or invaginations, of the plasma membrane that extend into the depths of the muscle fiber. These invaginations, called the transverse tubule system, are illustrated in Figure 9-10. The long fingers of plasma membrane projecting into the cell provide a path for depolarization resulting from an action potential in the surface membrane to influence events in the interior of the cell.

In most animal species, the transverse tubules occur just at the boundary between the A band and the I band. At locations where the transverse tubule encounters the sarcoplasmic reticulum, the membranes come into close apposition to form a structure called a triad. This is presumably the point of interaction between the depolarizing signal and the membrane of the sarcoplasmic reticulum. Note, however, that although the membranes are close together at a triad, they do not touch. Because the membranes are not in continuity, the depolarization produced during the action

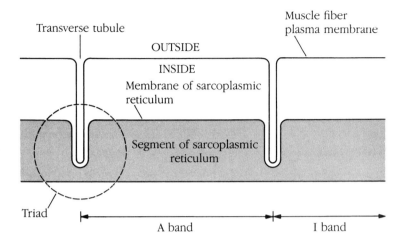

Transverse tubule

OUTSIDE

INSIDE

Membrane of sarcoplasmic
reticulum

Muscle fiber
plasma membrane

Segment of sarcoplasmic
reticulum

Triad

A band | I band

Figure 9-10
The transverse tubules are invaginations of the plasma membrane of the muscle fiber. Depolarization during an action potential can spread along the transverse tubules to the interior of the fiber. The triad is a region where the membranes of the tubule and the sarcoplasmic reticulum come into close proximity, and presumably represents the area where depolarization acts to release calcium from the sarcoplasmic reticulum.

potential cannot spread directly to the sarcoplasmic reticulum. Therefore, some indirect signal is required to link depolarization of the transverse tubule to calcium release by the sarcoplasmic reticulum.

Because calcium release from the sarcoplasmic reticulum is mediated via channels that are themselves activated by an increase in cytoplasmic calcium concentration, it is natural to suppose that the link between transverse tubules and sarcoplasmic reticulum is mediated by an influx of calcium ions from the extracellular space. Indeed, there are voltage-dependent calcium channels in the membrane of the transverse tubules that are opened by depolarization, and these calcium channels are required for the initiation of contraction. In cardiac muscle, an influx of calcium from the ECF via these depolarization-activated calcium channels is in fact required to initiate the muscle contraction, so that calcium ions through the transverse tubule calcium channels do indeed trigger the calcium release from the sarcoplasmic reticulum. However, in skeletal muscle, calcium influx via the calcium channels of the transverse tubules is not required to trigger contraction; some other linkage mechanism is required. The mechanism is not yet understood in detail, but it is thought that the calcium channels of the transverse tubule act as voltage sensors to detect the depolarization produced by the action potential and that there is a direct physical link, extending through the intracellular space, connecting single calcium-induced calcium release channels in the sarcoplasmic reticulum membrane to single voltage-dependent calcium channels in the immediately adjacent membrane of the transverse tubule. Perhaps conformation changes in the trans-

verse tubule calcium channel upon depolarization induce conformation changes in the calcium-induced calcium release channels
via this physical linkage, causing the local release of calcium from
the sarcoplasmic reticulum and initiating the explosive calcium-
induced release of calcium from the sarcoplasmic reticulum as a
whole.

Summary

The sequence of events leading to the contraction of a skeletal
muscle fiber following stimulation of its motor neuron can be
summarized as follows:

1. Acetylcholine released from the presynaptic terminal depolarizes the end-plate region of the muscle fiber.
2. The depolarization initiates an all-or-none action potential
in the muscle fiber, and the action potential propagates
along the entire length of the fiber.
3. Depolarization produced by the action potential spreads to
the interior of the fiber along the transverse tubule system.
4. Depolarization of the transverse tubules causes the release
of calcium ions by the sarcoplasmic reticulum.
5. Released calcium ions bind to troponin molecules on the
thin filaments.
6. When calcium combines with troponin, tropomyosin uncovers the myosin binding site of actin.
7. Globular heads of myosin molecules, which have been energized by splitting a high-energy phosphate bond of ATP,
are then free to bind to actin.
8. The stored energy of the activated myosin is released to propel the thick and thin filaments past each other. The spent
ADP is released from myosin at this point.
9. A new ATP binds to myosin, releasing its attachment to the
actin molecule.
10. The new ATP is split to re-energize myosin and return the
contraction cycle to step 7 above.
11. Contraction is maintained as long as the internal calcium
concentration is elevated. The calcium concentration falls as
calcium ions are taken back into the sarcoplasmic reticulum
via an ATP-dependent calcium pump.

Contraction of
Whole Muscle

Up to this point, we have been concerned with the physiology of muscle at the level of single muscle fibers. We have come to some understanding of the mechanisms involved in the linkage between an action potential in a presynaptic motor neuron and the contraction of the postsynaptic muscle cell. We learned that the motor neuron depolarizes the muscle fiber, causing an action potential that, in turn, triggers the all-or-none contraction of the fiber. At this point, we step back a bit from this cellular perspective and look at the functioning of a skeletal muscle as a whole. We consider how the all-or-none twitches of single muscle fibers are integrated into the smooth, graded movements we know our muscles are capable of making.

The Motor Unit

A single motor neuron makes synaptic contact with a number of muscle fibers. The actual number varies considerably from one muscle to another and from one motor neuron to another within the same muscle; a single motor neuron may contact as few as 10 to 20 muscle fibers or more than 1000. However, in mammals, a single muscle fiber normally receives synaptic contact from only one motor neuron. Therefore, a single motor neuron and the muscle fibers to which it is connected form a basic unit of motor organization called the **motor unit**. A schematic diagram of the organization of a motor unit is shown in Figure 10-1. Recall from Chapter 7 that the synapse between a motor neuron and a mus-

Figure 10-1
Schematic illustration of the innervation of a small number of muscle fibers in a muscle. The shaded muscle fibers form part of the motor unit of motor neuron 1 and the unshaded fibers form part of the motor unit of motor neuron 2.

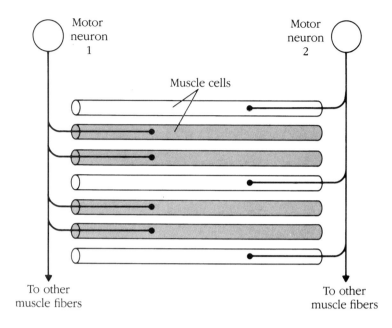

cle fiber is a one-for-one synapse—that is, a single presynaptic action potential produces a single postsynaptic action potential and hence a single twitch of the muscle cell. This means, then, that all the muscle cells in a motor unit contract together and that the fundamental unit of contraction of the whole muscle will not be the contraction of a single muscle fiber, but the contraction produced by all the muscle cells in a motor unit.

Gradation in the overall strength with which a particular muscle contracts is under control of the nervous system. There are two basic ways the nervous system uses to accomplish this task: (1) variation in the total number of motor neurons activated, and hence in the total number of motor units contracting; and (2) variation in the frequency of action potentials in the motor neuron of a single motor unit. The greater the number of motor units activated, the greater the strength of contraction; similarly, within limits, the greater the rate of action potentials within a motor unit, the greater the strength of the resulting summed contraction. We consider each of these mechanisms in turn below.

The Mechanics of Contraction

When the nerve controlling a muscle is stimulated, the resulting action potentials in the muscle fibers set up the sliding interaction between the filaments of the individual myofibrils in the muscle. This sliding generates a force that tends to make the muscle fibers, and therefore the muscle as a whole, shorten. Whether or not the muscle actually shortens, however, depends on the load attached to the muscle. While we might attempt to order the muscles in our arms to lift an automobile, it is unlikely that the muscles would be able to shorten against such a load. The force developed in an activated muscle is called the muscle **tension**, and only if the tension is great enough to equal the weight of the load will the muscle shorten and lift the load.

We can distinguish between two kinds of responses to activation of a muscle. If the muscle tension is less than the load, the contraction is said to be **isometric** ("same length") because the length of the muscle does not change even though the tension increases. That is, the force exerted on the load by the muscle is not sufficient to move the load, so the muscle cannot shorten. An isometric contraction is diagrammed in Figure 10-2A. In the figure, an isolated muscle is attached to a load it cannot lift. When the muscle is activated, the resulting tension is registered by a strain gauge that measures the minuscule flexing of the rigid strut to which the muscle is attached. A single activation of the muscle triggers a transient increase in tension lasting typically about 0.1 second. You can easily feel the tension developed in an isometric contraction by placing your palms together with your arms flexed in front of your chest and pushing with both hands, one against the other.

If the tension is great enough to overcome the weight of the load, the contraction is said to be **isotonic** ("same tension") because the tension remains constant once it reaches the level necessary to move the load. This situation is diagrammed in Figure 10-2B. The strain gauge again records the increase in tension, as with the isometric contraction. When the tension reaches the level necessary to lift the load, it levels off and the muscle begins to shorten as the load is lifted. During the change in muscle length, the tension remains constant and equal to the weight of the load. This is because it is this weight—hanging from the muscle and support strut—that determines the flexing measured by the strain gauge. Thus, while the muscle is changing length, the contraction is isotonic. In an isotonic contraction, the force developed by the sliding filaments in the myofibrils making up the muscle produces work in the form of moving the load through space.

One difference between isometric and isotonic contractions can be seen in the different delays between muscle activation

(A)

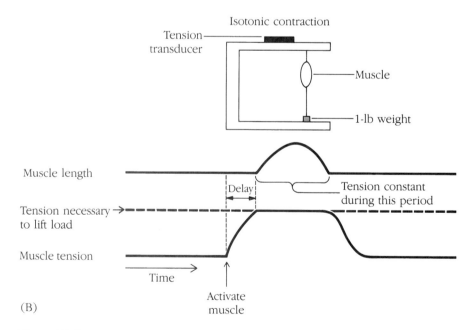

(B)

Figure 10-2
Measures of muscle length and muscle tension during (A) isometric and (B) isotonic contractions. At the upward arrow, the nerve innervating the muscle is stimulated, causing activation of the muscle fibers.

and the occurrence of a measurable change in either muscle tension (isometric) or muscle length (isotonic). The tension begins to rise within a few milliseconds, the time required for the effect of the excitation-contraction process discussed in Chapter 9 to take hold. However, if muscle length is measured instead, there is a pronounced delay between activation of the muscle and beginning of shortening. This delay is the time required for the tension to rise to the point where the load is lifted, which will depend on the size of the load. Thus, with light loads the shortening begins quickly, but with heavier loads the onset of shortening is progressively delayed. Finally, with sufficiently heavy loads there is no shortening at all and the contraction becomes isometric. In addition, with heavier loads the duration of shortening will be less and the maximum speed of shortening will be slower. In a sense, the measurement of tension during an isometric contraction gives a more direct view of the contractile state of the muscle; for this reason, subsequent examples in this chapter are of isometric contractions.

The Relationship Between Isometric Tension and Muscle Length

At this point, it is worth considering how the magnitude of the isometric tension developed by a muscle depends on the muscle length at which the tension is measured; this will allow us to relate the tension of the muscle as a whole to the microscopic contractile apparatus within each muscle fiber and to the sliding filament hypothesis discussed in Chapter 9. Suppose the experiment diagrammed in Figure 10-2A were repeated at a variety of lengths of the muscle, as set by varying the distance between the upper support bar and the weight. We would find that as the muscle is stretched beyond its normal resting length, the tension developed upon stimulating the muscle would fall off rapidly, falling to zero at about 175% of resting length. This is shown in Figure 10-3A, in which peak isometric tension is plotted against muscle length (expressed as a percentage of the resting length of the unstimulated muscle). Such behavior can be easily understood in terms of the underlying state of the thick and thin filaments making up each sarcomere. As the distance between Z lines increases, the degree of overlap between thick and thin filaments declines, and thus the number of myosin head groups available to form crossbridges is reduced. Finally, with sufficient stretch, there is no

Figure 10-3
The relation between muscle length and strength of isometric tension. (A) This graph shows the relation between isometric tension developed when a muscle is stimulated, expressed as a percentage of the maximum observed, and the length of the muscle, expressed as a percentage of resting length. The shaded area shows the range of muscle length over which the muscle would actually operate in the body. (B) These diagrams show the states of the thick and thin filaments within a sarcomere at each of the three numbered positions marked in (A).

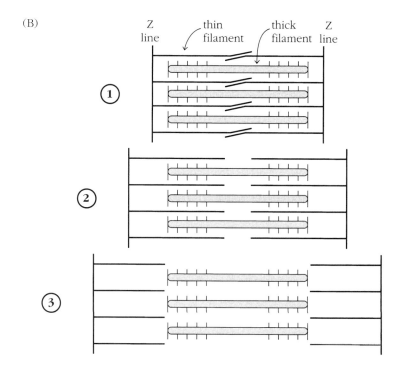

overlap, as shown in Figure 10-3B (number 3), and no tension can be developed.

If the muscle is artificially shortened, isometric tension is also reduced, falling to zero at about 50% of resting length. This effect occurs as the distance between successive Z lines becomes sufficiently short that there is overlap between the thin filaments attached to neighboring Z lines. This overlap distorts the necessary spatial relation between thin and thick filaments required for cross-bridge attachments to form, so that once again there are fewer cross-bridges available to develop tension, as shown in Figure 10-3B (number 1). In addition to this geometrical effect, other factors (such as reduced coupling between depolarization of the membrane and release of calcium from the sarcoplasmic reticulum) might contribute to the reduced peak tension at short muscle lengths. The fall-off of tension with both increasing and decreasing length means that there is an optimal range of length for the development of tension; in this optimal range, there is maximal overlap of thin filaments with the cross-bridges of the thick filament (Figure 10-3B, number 2). If a muscle is to operate at maximum efficiency, the range of length over which it is required to develop force when in actual use in the body should be close to this optimal range. This is indeed the case; as a skeletal muscle operates, its length remains within about 30% of the optimal length (the shaded region in Figure 10-3A). In order to ensure that this range is not exceeded, precise arrangements of muscle fiber length, tendon length and attachment sites, and joint geometry have evolved to be appropriate for the functional task of each muscle.

Control of Muscle Tension by the Nervous System

Recruitment of Motor Neurons

A single muscle typically receives inputs from hundreds of motor neurons. Thus, tension in the muscle can be increased by increasing the number of these motor neurons that are firing action potentials; the tension produced by activating individual motor units sums to produce the total tension in the muscle. A simplified example is shown in Figure 10-4. The increase in the number of active motor neurons is called **recruitment** of motor neurons and is an important physiological means of controlling muscle tension.

Figure 10-4

A simple muscle consisting of four motor units of varying size. The graph (bottom) shows isometric tension in response to simultaneous action potentials (at the arrow) in various combinations of the motor neurons.

Motor neurons

Muscle fibers

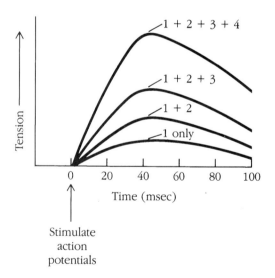

When motor neurons are recruited into action during naturally oc-curring motor behavior, such as locomotion or lifting loads, the order of recruitment is determined by the size of the motor unit. As the tension in a muscle is increased, starting from the relaxed state, motor units containing a small number of muscle fibers are the first to be recruited; larger motor units are recruited later.

Figure 10-5

Comparison of speed of development of isometric tension in fast and slow muscle fibers.

Thus, when there is little activity in the pool of motor neurons controlling a muscle and the tension in the muscle is low, small motor units are recruited to produce an increase in tension. This ensures that the added increments of tension are small, and prevents large jerky increases in tension when the tension is low. As tension increases, however, further increases in tension must be larger in order to make a significant difference; thus, larger motor units are added, resulting in larger increments of tension when the background tension is already high. This behavior is referred to as the **size principle** in motor neuron recruitment. In Figure 10-4, for example, it would be expected that tension would be increased by adding the smaller motor units (numbers 1 and 2) first and the largest unit (number 4) last.

Fast and Slow Muscle Fibers

The time delay between the occurrence of the muscle fiber action potential and the peak of the resulting tension is not constant across all muscle fibers. The delay to peak tension can be as little as 10 or as many as 200 msec. In general, muscle fibers can be grouped into two classes—fast and slow—on the basis of this speed. Samples of isometric contractions in fast and slow fibers are shown in Figure 10-5. Both slow and fast fibers are found together in most muscles, but slow fibers predominate in muscles that must maintain steady contraction, such as those involved in keeping us standing upright. Fast muscle fibers are more common in muscles that require rapid contraction, such as those involved in jumping and running. The fastest muscle fibers are those of muscles that move the eyes in rapid jumps, like those your eyes are making as you scan the words on this page.

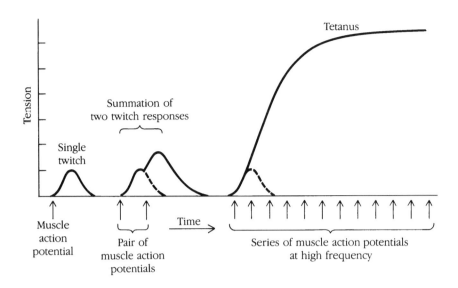

Figure 10-6

Isometric tension in response to a series of action potentials in a muscle. The dashed lines show the expected response if only the first action potential of a series occurred.

Temporal Summation of Contractions Within a Single Motor Unit

When motor neurons are activated during naturally occurring movement, they do not typically fire just a single action potential, as has been the case in all our examples so far. Rather, action potentials tend to occur in bursts of several discharges or as steady discharges at a relatively constant frequency. It is not uncommon for action potentials within a burst to be separated by only 10 msec or less. Under normal conditions, each of these many action potentials in a motor neuron will produce a corresponding action potential in each of the motor unit's muscle fibers. Because the tension resulting from a single action potential typically lasts for many tens or hundreds of milliseconds, there is considerable opportunity for summation of the effects of succeeding muscle action potentials in a series, as illustrated in Figure 10-6. Such temporal summation of individual twitches is a major way the nervous system controls tension in skeletal muscles.

The amount of summation within a burst of muscle action potentials depends on the frequency of action potentials: The higher the frequency, the greater the resulting summed tension. However, as shown in Figure 10-6, when the frequency is sufficiently high, the individual tension responses of the muscle fuse together into a plateau of tension. A further increase in frequency beyond this point does not increase tension: The muscle has reached its maximum response and cannot develop further tension. This plateau state is called **tetanus**. As expected from the examples shown in Figure 10-5, the frequency of stimulation required to produce tetanus varies considerably depending on whether slow or fast fibers are involved. For fast fibers, a frequency of more than 100 action potentials per second may be required, while for slow fibers a frequency of 20 per second may suffice.

Asynchronous Activation of Motor Units During Maintained Contraction

As anyone who has done prolonged physical labor or exercised vigorously can attest, muscle contractions cannot be maintained indefinitely; muscles fatigue and must be rested. Thus, the state of tetanus depicted in Figure 10-6 could not be maintained in a single motor unit for very long without allowing the muscle fibers in the motor unit to relax. However, some muscles, such as those involved in maintaining body posture, are required to contract for prolonged periods. What mechanism helps prevent muscle fatigue during such prolonged contractions? During maintained tension in a muscle, all the motor neurons to the muscle are not active at the same time. The activity of the motor units occurs in bursts separated by quiet periods, and the activity of different motor units is staggered in time. An example of this kind of asynchronous activity during steady contraction is shown in Figure 10-7. Notice that the summation of the tensions produced by the activity of only three motor units, each active only half the time, can produce a reasonably smooth, steady tension. With hundreds of motor units available in many muscles, a much smoother and larger steady tension could be maintained with less effort on the part of any one motor unit. Thus, asynchronous activation of motor neurons to a muscle allows a prolonged contraction with reduced fatigue of individual motor units in the muscle.

Summary

The basic unit of contraction of a skeletal muscle is the contraction of the group of muscle fibers making up a single motor unit, which consists of a single motor neuron and all the muscle fibers receiving synaptic connections from that neuron. Whenever the motor neuron fires an action potential, all the muscle fibers in that motor unit twitch together. The magnitude of the contraction gen-

Figure 10-7

Summation of muscle tension
during asynchronous activation
of three motor units in a muscle.

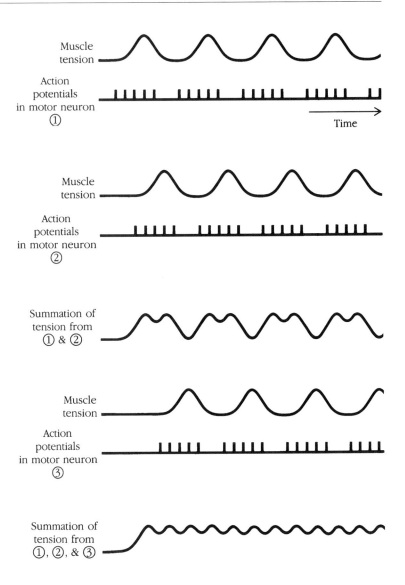

erated by activation of a motor unit depends on the number of
muscle fibers in that motor unit. The number of fibers in a unit,
and hence the magnitude of the tension produced by activating
the unit, varies considerably among the set of motor neurons innervating a particular muscle.

The type of contraction produced by activation of a whole muscle depends on the load against which the muscle is contracting.
If the load is too great for the muscle to move, the length of the
muscle does not change during the contraction, which is then
called an isometric contraction. If the tension is sufficient to over-

come the weight of the load, the contraction will be accompanied by a shortening of the muscle. During the shortening, the tension in the muscle remains constant and equal to the weight of the load. Such a contraction is called isotonic. The overall tension developed by a muscle depends on how many motor units are activated and on the frequency of action potentials within a motor unit. Increasing muscle tension by increasing the number of active motor neurons is called motor neuron recruitment. When the frequency of action potentials within a motor unit is increased, the resulting muscle tension increases until a steady plateau state, called tetanus, is reached. Normally, during a maintained contraction all the motor neurons of a muscle are not active simultaneously; rather, the activity of individual motor neurons is restricted to periodic bursts that occur asynchronously among the pool of motor neurons controlling a muscle. This helps reduce fatigue in the muscle by allowing individual motor units to rest periodically during a maintained contraction.

11

Cardiac Muscle: The Autonomic Nervous System

The motor functions we have described so far in this part of the book concern the control of skeletal muscles. These are the muscles that produce overt movements of the body and give rise to the observable external actions that we normally think of as the "behavior" of an animal. However, even in an animal that appears to an external observer to be quiescent, the nervous system is quite busy coordinating many ongoing motor actions that are as important for survival as skeletal muscle movements. These motor activities include regulating digestion, maintaining the proper glucose balance in the blood, regulating heart rate, and so on. The part of the nervous system that controls these functions is called the **autonomic nervous system**. The motor targets of the autonomic nervous system include gland cells, cardiac muscle cells, and smooth muscle cells such as those found in the gut. To distinguish them from the autonomic nervous system, the parts of the nervous system we have been discussing up to this point— whose motor targets are the skeletal muscles—are collectively called the **somatic nervous system**.

In addition to the differences in their target cells, there are other differences between the autonomic and somatic nervous systems. As we have learned, in the somatic nervous system, the cell bodies of the motor neurons are located within the central nervous system, either in the spinal cord or in the nuclei of cranial nerves in the brainstem. By contrast, the cell bodies of the motor neurons in the autonomic nervous system are located outside the central nervous system altogether, in a system of autonomic ganglia distributed throughout the body. The central nervous system controls these autonomic ganglia by way of output neurons called preganglionic neurons, which are located in the spinal cord and brainstem. This arrangement is illustrated in Figure 11-1. The motor neurons in the autonomic ganglia are also called postganglionic neurons. The axons of the preganglionic neurons entering the ganglia are referred to as the preganglionic fibers, while the axons of the autonomic motor neurons carrying the output to the target cells are called the postganglionic fibers. Thus, in the somatic nervous system, the motor commands exiting from the central nervous system go directly to the target cells, while in the autonomic nervous system, the motor commands from the central nervous system are relayed via an additional synaptic connection in the peripheral nervous system.

The autonomic and somatic nervous systems also differ in the effects that the motor neurons have on the target cells. In Chapter 7, we discussed in detail the synaptic interaction between motor neurons and skeletal muscle cells at the neuromuscular junction. All of the somatic motor neurons release acetylcholine as their neurotransmitter, and the effect on the skeletal muscle cells is always excitatory: Contraction is stimulated. In the autonomic nervous system, however, some motor neurons release acetylcholine and other motor neurons release the neurotransmitter norepinephrine (see Chapter 8), instead of acetylcholine. Further, an autonomic motor neuron may either excite or inhibit its target cell. In general, if norepinephrine excites the target cells, then acetylcholine inhibits them, and vice versa. For example, norepinephrine increases the rate of beating of the heart, while acetylcholine decreases the heart rate, as we will examine in detail shortly.

The norepinephrine-releasing and acetylcholine-releasing motor neurons are organized into anatomically distinct divisions of the autonomic nervous system, called the **sympathetic division** (norepinephrine releasing) and the **parasympathetic division** (acetylcholine releasing). The ganglia containing the sympathetic motor neurons are called sympathetic ganglia, and those containing parasympathetic motor neurons are called parasympathetic ganglia. Most of the sympathetic ganglia are arrayed parallel to the spinal cord, one ganglion on each side just outside the vertebral column. There is one pair of these paravertebral ganglia for each vertebral segment. The ganglia are interconnected by thick, longitudinal bundles of axons containing the preganglionic fibers exiting from the spinal cord. Because of these connectives, the paravertebral ganglia form two long chains parallel to the spinal column, sometimes referred to as the sympathetic chains. In addition to the

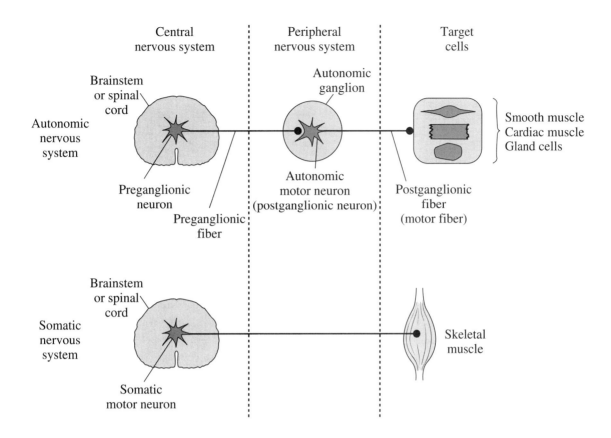

Figure 11-1

Differences between autonomic and somatic nervous systems. In the autonomic nervous system, the motor neurons are located outside the central nervous system, in autonomic ganglia. The motor neurons contact smooth muscle cells, cardiac muscle cells, and gland cells. The central nervous system controls the ganglia via preganglionic neurons. In the somatic nervous system, the motor neurons are located within the central nervous system and contact skeletal muscle cells.

paravertebral ganglia that make up the chains, there also are sympathetic ganglia called the prevertebral ganglia, located within the abdomen.

The parasympathetic ganglia are distributed more diffusely throughout the body and tend to be located closer to their target organs. In some cases, the parasympathetic ganglia are actually located within the target organ itself. This is the case, for example, in the heart. Because the sympathetic ganglia are located predominantly near the central nervous system while the parasympathetic ganglia are located mostly near to their target organs, the preganglionic fibers of the sympathetic nervous system are usually much shorter than the preganglionic fibers of the parasympathetic nervous system, which must extend all the way from the central nervous system to the near vicinity of the target organ in order to reach the postganglionic neurons. Conversely, the postganglionic fibers are typically much longer in the sympathetic nervous system than in the parasympathetic nervous system.

Most target organs receive inputs from both the sympathetic and parasympathetic divisions of the autonomic nervous system. As noted already, the sympathetic and parasympathetic inputs produce opposing effects on the target. In general, excitation of the sympathetic nervous system has the overall effect of placing the organism in "emergency mode," ready for vigorous activity. The parasympathetic nervous system has the opposite effect of placing the organism in a "vegetative mode." For example, sympathetic activity increases the heart rate and blood pressure, diverts blood flow from the skin and viscera to the skeletal muscles, and reduces intestinal motility, all appropriate preparations for rapid reaction to an external threat. Parasympathetic activity, on the other hand, decreases heart rate and blood pressure, and promotes blood circulation to the gut and intestinal motility. All of these actions are appropriate for resting and digesting, in the absence of any threatening situation in the environment.

To see how the motor neurons of the sympathetic and parasympathetic divisions exert their actions on target cells, it will be useful to examine a particular example in detail. The example we explore is the neural control of the heart. The heart is made up of muscle cells that are in some ways similar to the skeletal muscle cells we learned about in Chapter 9. However, there are some important differences that we must understand before we can examine the effects that the sympathetic and parasympathetic neurons have on the heart. Thus, we first discuss the electrical and mechanical properties of the heart muscle, and then return to the modulation of these properties by norepinephrine and acetylcholine, which are the neurotransmitters released by the sympathetic and parasympathetic inputs to the heart, respectively.

The Pattern of Cardiac Contraction

Cardiac muscle cells contain a contractile apparatus like that of other striated muscle, being made up of bundles of myofilaments with a microscopic structure like that discussed in Chapter 9. Unlike other striated muscles in the body, the heart muscle is specialized to produce a rhythmic and coordinated contraction in order to drive the blood efficiently through the blood vessels. The heart has a number of tasks to accomplish in order to carry out its role in providing oxygen to the cells of the body. It must receive the oxygen-poor blood returning from the body tissues via the venous circulation and send that blood to the lungs for oxygenation. It must also receive the oxygenated blood from the lungs and send it out through the arterial circulation to the rest of the body. Carrying out these tasks requires precise timing of the contractions of the various heart chambers; otherwise, the flow of oxygenated blood will not occur efficiently or will cease altogether—with disastrous consequences. What is the normal timing sequence of the heart contractions underlying the coordinated pumping of the blood?

A schematic diagram of the flow of blood through a human heart during a single contraction cycle is shown in Figure 11-2. Humans, like all other mammals, have a four-chambered heart, consisting of the left and right atria and the left and right ventricles. The two atria can be thought of as the receiving chambers, or "priming" pumps, of the heart, while the two ventricles are the "power" pumps of the circulatory system. The right atrium receives the blood returning from the body through the veins, and the left atrium receives the freshly oxygenated blood from the lungs. During the phase of the heartbeat when the atria are filling with blood, the valves connecting the atria with the ventricles are closed, preventing the flow of blood into the ventricles. When the atria have filled with blood, they contract and the increase in pressure opens the valves leading to the ventricles and drives the collected blood into the ventricles. At this point, the muscle of the ventricles is relaxed, and the valves connecting the ventricles to the vessels leaving the heart are closed. When the ventricles have filled with blood, they contract, opening these valves and delivering the power stroke to drive the blood out to the lungs and to the rest of the body, as shown in Figure 11-2B. Thus, during a normal heartbeat the two atria contract together, followed after a delay by the simultaneous contraction of the two ventricles.

Coordination of Contraction Across Cardiac Muscle Fibers

In order for the contraction of a heart chamber to be able to propel the expulsion of fluid, all the individual muscle fibers making up the walls of that chamber must contract together. It is this unified contraction that constricts the cavity of the chamber and drives the blood out into the blood vessels of the circulation. In skeletal muscles, an action potential in one muscle fiber is confined to that fiber and does not influence neighboring fibers; therefore,

Figure 11-2
Schematic drawings of the state of the heart valves and the direction of blood flow during two stages in a single heartbeat. (A) The atria are contracting and the ventricles are filling with blood. (B) The valves between the atria and ventricles are closed and the ventricles are contracting, forcing the blood out to the lungs (right ventricle) and to the arteries leading to the rest of the body (left ventricle).

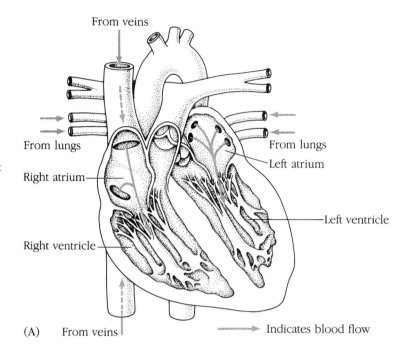

From veins

From lungs

Right atrium

Right ventricle

From lungs

Left atrium

Left ventricle

(A)   From veins

⟶ Indicates blood flow

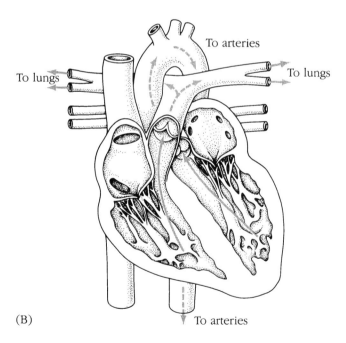

To arteries

To lungs

To lungs

(B)

To arteries

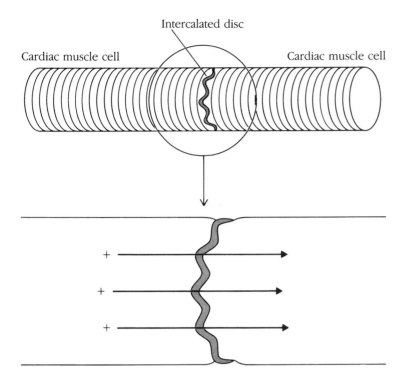

Intercalated disc

Cardiac muscle cell   Cardiac muscle cell

Figure 11-3
Electrical current can flow from one cardiac muscle cell to another through specialized membrane junctions located in a region of contact called the intercalated disc.

contraction is restricted to the particular fiber undergoing an action potential. In cardiac muscle, however, the situation is quite different. When an action potential is generated in a cardiac muscle fiber, it causes action potentials in the neighboring fibers, which in turn set up action potentials in their neighbors, and so on. Thus, the excitation spreads rapidly out through all the muscle fibers of the chamber. This ensures that all the fibers contract together.

What characteristic of cardiac muscle fibers allows the action potential to spread from one fiber to another? This can be seen by looking at the microscopic structure of the cells of cardiac muscle, as shown schematically in Figure 11-3. At the ends of each cardiac cell, the plasma membranes of neighboring cells come into close contact at specialized structures called intercalated discs. The contact at this point is sufficiently close that electrical current flowing inside one fiber can cross directly into the interior of the next fiber; in electrical terms, it is as though the neighboring cells form one larger cell. Recall from Chapter 5 that an electrical current flowing along the interior of a fiber has at each point two paths to choose from: across the plasma membrane or

Figure 11-4
An experiment in which the membrane potentials of two cells are measured simultaneously with intracellular microelectrodes. (A) A depolarizing current is injected into cell 1. (B) If the cells are not electrically coupled, the depolarization occurs only in the cell in which the current was injected. (C) If the cells are electrically coupled via gap junctions, a depolarization occurs in cell 2, as well as in cell 1.

(A) Experimental arrangement

(B) Cells not coupled

(C) Cells electrically coupled

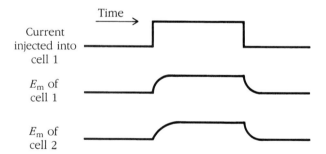

along the interior of the fiber. The amount of current taking each path at a particular point depends on the relative resistances of the two paths; the higher the resistance, the smaller the amount of current taking that path. Normally, at the point where one cell ends and the next begins, there is little opportunity for current to flow from one cell to the other because the current would have to flow out across one cell membrane and in across the other in order to do so; this is a high-resistance path because current must cross two membranes. At the specialized structure of the intercalated disc, however, the resistance to current flow across the two membranes is low, so that the path to the interior of the neighboring cell is favored. This means that depolarizing current in-jected into one cell during the occurrence of an action potential can spread directly into neighboring cells, setting up an action po-tential in those cells as well. The low-resistance path from one cell to another is through membrane structures called **gap junc-tions**. These structures consist of arrays of small pores directly connecting the interiors of the joined cells, so that small mole-cules like ions can pass directly from one cell to another.

When electrical current can pass from one cell to another, as in cardiac muscle, those cells are said to be **electrically coupled**. An electrophysiological experiment to demonstrate this behavior is illustrated in Figure 11-4. When current is injected into a cell, no response occurs in a neighboring cell if the cells are not electrically coupled. If the two cells are coupled via gap junctions, a response to the injected current occurs in both cells because the ions carrying the current inside the cell can pass directly through the gap junction. If the depolarization is large enough, an action potential will be triggered in both cells at the same time.

Generation of Rhythmic Contractions

The electrical coupling among cardiac muscle fibers can explain how contraction occurs synchronously in all the fibers of a cham-ber. We now consider the control mechanisms responsible for the repetitive contractions that characterize the beating of the heart. If a heart is removed from the body and placed in an appropri-ate artificial environment, the heart muscles will continue to con-tract repetitively even though they are isolated from the nervous system and the rest of the body. In contrast, a skeletal muscle iso-lated under similar conditions will not contract unless its nerve is activated. The rhythmic activity of the heart muscle is an inherent property of the individual muscle fibers making up the heart, and this constitutes another important difference between cardiac muscle fibers and skeletal muscle fibers. This difference can be demonstrated dramatically in experiments in which muscle tissue is dissociated into individual cells, which are placed in a dish iso-lated from each other and from the influence of any other cells, like nerve cells. Under these conditions, muscle cells from skele-tal muscles are quiescent; they do not contract in the absence of their neural input. Cells from cardiac muscle, however, continue to contract rhythmically even in isolation. Thus, rhythmic contrac-tions of heart muscle are due to built-in properties of the cardiac muscle cells. Before we can examine the membrane mechanism underlying this **autorhythmicity**, it is necessary to look first at the action potential of cardiac muscle cells. In keeping with the different behavior of cardiac cells, this action potential has some different characteristics from the action potentials of neurons or skeletal muscle cells.

The Cardiac Action Potential

In Chapters 5 and 6, we discussed the ionic mechanisms underlying the action potential of nerve membrane. The action potential of skeletal muscle fibers is fundamentally the same as that of neurons. The cardiac action potential, however, is different from these other action potentials in several important ways. Figure 11-5 compares the characteristics of action potentials of skeletal and cardiac muscle cells. One striking difference is the difference in time scale: Cardiac action potentials can last several hundred milliseconds, while skeletal muscle action potentials are typically over in 1 to 2 msec. As we learned in Chapter 5, a long-lasting plateau like that of the cardiac action potential can arise from a calcium component in the action potential, resulting from the opening of voltage-dependent calcium channels. These channels open upon depolarization and allow the influx of positively charged calcium ions. In addition, the plateau of the cardiac action potential is also associated with a reduction in the potassium permeability. This is due to a type of potassium channel that is open as long as the membrane potential is near its normal resting level and *closes* upon depolarization. This is the reverse of the behavior of the gated potassium channel we are familiar with from our discussion of nerve action potential. The reduction in potassium permeability caused by the closing of this channel tends to depolarize the cardiac muscle fiber. Both the opening of the calcium channels and the closing of the potassium channels contribute to the plateau.

The initial rising phase of the cardiac action potential is produced by voltage-dependent sodium channels very much like those of nerve membrane. The sodium channels drive the rapid initial depolarization and are responsible for the brief initial spike of the cardiac action potential before the plateau phase sets in. Like the sodium channel of neuronal membrane, this channel rapidly closes (inactivates) with maintained depolarization. However, unlike the nerve sodium channel, this inactivation is not total;

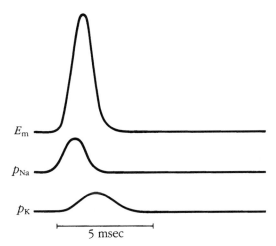

E_m

p_{Na}

p_K

5 msec

(A)   Skeletal muscle

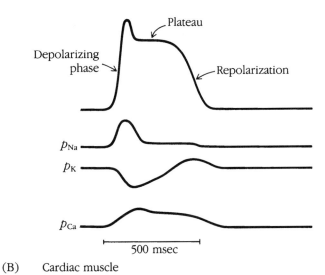

Plateau

Depolarizing
phase

Repolarization

p_{Na}

p_K

p_{Ca}

500 msec

(B)   Cardiac muscle

Figure 11-5
The sequence of permeability
changes underlying the action
potentials of (A) skeletal muscle
fibers and (B) cardiac muscle
fibers. Note the greatly different
time scales.

there is a small, maintained increase in sodium permeability during the plateau.

What is responsible for terminating the cardiac action potential? First, the calcium permeability of the plasma membrane slowly declines during the maintained depolarization. This decline might be a consequence of the gradual buildup of internal calcium concentration as calcium ions continue to enter the muscle fiber through the open calcium channels. Internal calcium ions are thought to have a direct or indirect action on the calcium channels, causing

Figure 11-6
(A) In a skeletal muscle fiber, the action potential is much briefer than the resulting contraction. Thus, the action potential acts only as a trigger for the contraction, which proceeds independently of the duration of the action potential. (B) In a cardiac muscle fiber, the duration of the contraction is closely related to the duration of the action potential because of the maintained calcium influx during the plateau of the action potential. Thus, characteristics of the action potential can influence the duration and strength of the cardiac contraction.

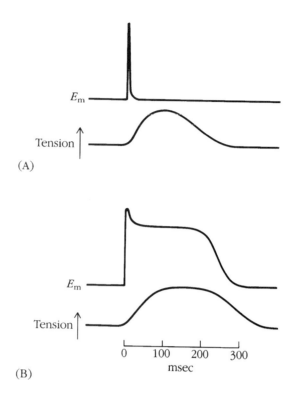

them to close. In addition, the potassium permeability of the plasma membrane increases, as in the nerve and skeletal muscle action potentials. This increase in potassium permeability tends to drive the membrane potential of the cardiac fiber toward the potassium equilibrium potential and thus to repolarize the fiber. There is evidence that part of this increase in potassium permeability is due to voltage-sensitive potassium channels that open in response to the depolarization during the action potential (like the *n* gates of the nerve membrane). However, the increased potassium permeability is also caused by calcium-activated potassium channels (see Chapter 5), which open in response to the rise in internal calcium concentration during the prolonged action potential.

One functional implication of the prolonged cardiac action potential is that the duration of the contraction in cardiac muscle is controlled by the duration of the action potential. The action potential and contraction of cardiac muscle fibers are compared with those of skeletal muscle fibers in Figure 11-6. In skeletal muscle, the action potential acts only as a trigger for the contractile events; the duration of the contraction is controlled by the timing of the release and reuptake of calcium by the sarcoplasmic reticulum, not by the duration of the action potential. In cardiac muscle fibers, however, only the initial part of the contraction is controlled by sarcoplasmic reticulum calcium; the contraction is maintained by the influx of calcium ions across the plasma membrane during the plateau phase of the cardiac action potential. For this reason, the duration of the contraction in the heart can be altered by changing the duration of the action potential in the cardiac muscle fibers. This provides an important mechanism by which the pumping action of the heart can be modulated.

The Pacemaker Potential

Although the ionic mechanism of the cardiac action potential differs in important ways from that of other action potentials, nothing in the scheme presented so far would account for the endogenous beating of isolated heart cells discussed earlier. If we recorded the electrical membrane potential of a spontaneously beating isolated heart cell, we would see a series of spontaneous action potentials, as shown in Figure 11-7. After each action potential, the potential falls to its normal negative resting value, then begins to depolarize slowly. This slow depolarization is called a **pacemaker potential**, and it is caused by spontaneous changes in the membrane ionic permeability. Voltage-clamp experiments on single isolated muscle fibers from the ventricles suggest that the pacemaker potential is due to a slow decline in the potassium permeability coupled with a slow increase in sodium and calcium permeability. When the depolarization reaches threshold, it triggers an action potential in the fiber, with a rapid upstroke caused by the opening of sodium channels and a prolonged plateau produced by calcium channels. Part of the early phase of the pacemaker potential represents the normal undershoot period of an action potential (see Chapter 5), when potassium channels that were opened by depolarization during the action potential slowly close again. As these potassium channels close, the membrane potential will move in a positive direction, away from the potassium equilibrium potential.

Later phases of the pacemaker potential represent increases in sodium and calcium permeability, both of which move the membrane potential in a more positive direction, toward the sodium and calcium equilibrium potentials. The sodium permeability increases during the pacemaker potential because of the opening of nonspecific cation channels, which open at more hyperpolar-

Figure 11-7
Recording of membrane potential during repetitive, spontaneous beating in a single cardiac muscle fiber. The repolarization at the end of one action potential is followed by a slow, spontaneous depolarization called the pacemaker potential. When this depolarization reaches threshold, a new action potential is triggered.

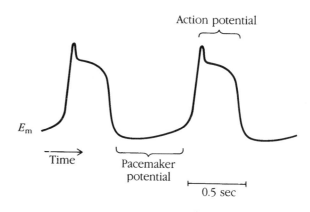

ized membrane potentials. As described in Chapter 7, the opening of channels with equal permeability to sodium and potassium ions (like the acetylcholine-activated channels at the neuromuscular junction) will produce depolarization of a cell. These hyperpolarization-activated cation channels are opened in response to the membrane hyperpolarization during the undershoot of the action potential. Together with the decrease in potassium permeability, the resulting influx of sodium ions moves the membrane potential of the cardiac cell in a positive direction, toward the threshold for firing an action potential. As the membrane potential becomes more positive during the pacemaker potential, voltage-dependent calcium channels open in response to the depolarization. The resulting influx of positively charged calcium ions produces even more depolarization, ultimately triggering the next action potential in the series.

The rate of spontaneous action potentials in isolated heart cells varies from one cell to another; some cells beat rapidly and others slowly. In the intact heart, however, the electrical coupling among the fibers guarantees that all the fibers will contract together, with the overall rate being governed by the fibers with the fastest pacemaker activity. In the normal functioning of the heart, the overall rate of beating is controlled by a special set of pacemaker cells, called the **sinoatrial (SA) node**, which is located in the upper part of the right atrium. This node is indicated in the diagram of the heart in Figure 11-8. The action potential of cells in the SA node is a bit different from that of other cardiac cells. In the SA node, calcium channels play a larger role than sodium channels in triggering the action potential, as well as in sustaining the depolarization during the action potential. In the normal resting human heart, the cells of the SA node generate spontaneous action potentials at a

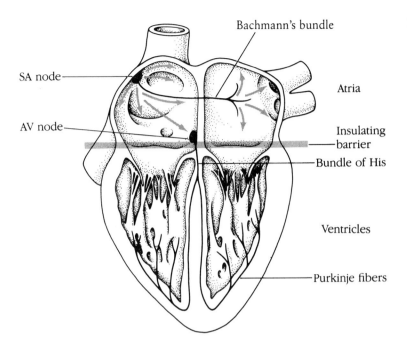

SA node

AV node

Bachmann's bundle

Atria

Insulating barrier

Bundle of His

Ventricles

Purkinje fibers

Figure 11-8
Diagram of the spread of action potentials across the heart during a single heartbeat. The excitation originates in the sinoatrial (SA) node of the right atrium and spreads throughout the atria via electrical coupling among the atrial muscle fibers. The spread is facilitated by special conducting fibers in Bachmann's bundle. The fibers of the atria are not electrically connected to those of the ventricles. The action potential spreads to the ventricles via the atrioventricular (AV) node, which introduces a delay between the atrial and ventricular action potentials. When the wave of action potentials leaves the AV node, its spread throughout the ventricles is aided by the rapidly conducting Purkinje fibers of the bundle of His.

rate of about 70 per minute. These action potentials spread through the electrical connections among fibers throughout the two atria, generating the simultaneous contraction of the atria as discussed in the first section of this chapter. The spread of excitation from the right to the left atrium is facilitated by a bundle of muscle fibers, called **Bachmann's bundle**, that are specialized for more rapid conduction of excitation. This helps ensure that the two atria contract together. The atrial action potentials do not spread directly to the fibers making up the two ventricles, however. This is a good thing, because we know that the contraction of the ventricles must be delayed to allow the relaxed ventricles to fill with blood pumped into them by the atrial contraction. In terms of electrical conduction, the heart behaves as two isolated units, as shown in Figure 11-8: The two atria are one unit and the two ventricles are another. The electrical connection between these two units is made via another specialized group of muscle fibers called the **atrioventricular (AV) node**. Excitation in the atria must travel through the AV node to reach the ventricles. The fibers of the AV node are small in diameter compared with other cardiac fibers. As discussed in Chapter 5, the speed of action potential conduction is slow in small-diameter fibers. Therefore, conduction through the AV node introduces a time delay sufficient to retard the contraction of the ventricles relative to the contraction of the atria. Excitation leaving the AV node does not travel directly through the muscle fibers of the ventricles. Instead, it travels along specialized muscle fibers that are designed for rapid conduction of action potentials. These fibers are called **Purkinje fibers**, and they form a fast-conducting pathway through the ventricles called the **bundle of His**. The Purkinje fibers carry the excitation rapidly to the apex at the base of the heart, where it then spreads out through the mass of ventricular muscle fibers to produce the contraction of the ventricles.

Actions of Acetylcholine and Norepinephrine on Cardiac Muscle Cells

Each muscle fiber of a skeletal muscle receives a direct synaptic input from a particular motor neuron; without this synaptic input, a skeletal muscle fiber does not contract unless stimulated directly by artificial means. On the other hand, we have seen that cardiac muscle fibers generate spontaneous contractions that are coordinated into a functional heartbeat by the electrical conduction mechanisms inherent in the heart itself. This does not mean, however, that the activity of the heart is not influenced by inputs from the nervous system. The heart receives two opposing neural inputs that affect the heart rate. One input comes from the cells of the parasympathetic nervous system, whose synaptic terminals in the heart release the neurotransmitter acetylcholine. The effect of acetylcholine is to slow the rate of depolarization during the pacemaker potential of the SA node. This has the effect of increasing the interval between successive action potentials and thus slowing the rate at which this master pacemaker region drives the heartbeat. Acetylcholine acts by increasing the potassium permeability of the muscle fiber membrane. This tends to keep the membrane potential closer to the potassium equilibrium potential and thus retard the growth of the pacemaker potential toward threshold for triggering an action potential. The second neural input to the heart comes from neurons of the sympathetic nervous system whose synaptic terminals release the neurotransmitter norepinephrine. Activation of this input speeds the heart rate and also increases the strength of contraction. This effect is mediated via an increase in the calcium permeability that is activated upon depolarization. Thus, the parasympathetic and sympathetic divisions of the autonomic nervous system have opposite effects on the heart, just as they typically do in all other target organs, as well.

Both the effect of acetylcholine on potassium channels and the effect of norepinephrine on calcium channels are indirect effects. Recall from Chapter 8 that neurotransmitters can affect ion channels either directly (as is the case for acetylcholine at the neuromuscular junction) or indirectly via intracellular second messengers. In the heart, the acetylcholine released by the parasympathetic neurons binds to and activates a type of acetylcholine receptor quite different from the nonspecific cation channel that is directly activated by acetylcholine at the neuromuscular junction. This type of receptor is called the **muscarinic acetylcholine receptor** (because it is activated by the drug muscarine and related compounds, as well as by acetylcholine). The acetylcholine receptor at the neuromuscular junction is called the nicotinic acetylcholine receptor (because it is activated by the drug nicotine and related compounds). Muscarinic receptors are not themselves ion channels. Instead, the activated receptor binds to and stimulates GTP binding proteins (G-proteins, see Chapter 8) that are attached to the inner surface of the membrane near the receptors. This sequence is diagrammed in Figure 11-9. In their active form, with GTP bound, the G-proteins then cause potassium channels to open, increasing the potassium permeability of the muscle cell and slowing the rate of action potentials. The effect of the G-proteins on the channel may be direct, by binding of the channel protein to one or more subunits of the active G-protein, or it may be indirect by stimulation of arachidonic acid, a second messenger produced by enzymatic cleavage of membrane lipids. The muscarinic receptor activates the G-protein by inducing the replacement of GDP by GTP at the GTP binding site. The G-protein remains active—interacting with and opening potassium channels—as long as GTP occupies the binding site on the G-protein. The activity of the G-protein is terminated by the intrinsic GTPase activity of the G-protein itself, which ultimately hydrolyzes the terminal phosphate of the GTP, converting it to the inactive GDP.

The linkage between the norepinephrine receptor of the cardiac muscle cells and the calcium channels is also mediated via G-proteins. This is summarized in Figure 11-10. The receptor on the cell surface that detects norepinephrine is a type called the **β-adrenergic receptor** (there is also a different class of norepinephrine receptor called the α-adrenergic receptor, but that class is not involved in the effects of norepinephrine we are discussing here).

Figure 11-9
Acetylcholine (ACh) indirectly opens potassium channels in cardiac muscle cells. Acetylcholine released from the synaptic terminals of parasympathetic neurons binds to a postsynaptic receptor, called a muscarinic acetylcholine receptor. When acetylcholine is bound, the receptor in turn activates G-proteins, by catalyzing the replacement of GDP by GTP on the GTP binding site of the G-protein. The activated G-protein, with GTP bound, then interacts either directly or indirectly with the potassium channel, causing the channel to open and allow an efflux of potassium ions. The G-protein has three subunits, as drawn, and GTP binds to only one of them, called the α-subunit. The other two subunits (β and γ) dissociate from the α-subunit when GTP binds, and it is thought that the β- and γ-subunits are the ones that actually interact with the potassium channels.

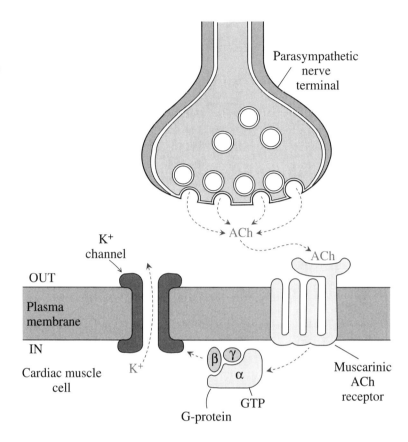

β-Adrenergic receptors are members of the same family of receptors as the muscarinic cholinergic receptors we just discussed. Like the muscarinic receptor, the β-adrenergic receptor is not itself an ion channel. The receptor activates G-proteins inside the cell when norepinephrine occupies its binding site on the outside of the cell. In this case in the heart, the G-protein is a member of a class that exerts its cellular actions by changing the level of cyclic AMP inside the cell. The synthetic enzyme for cyclic AMP, adenylyl cyclase, is activated by the G-protein, causing cyclic AMP levels to rise inside the cardiac cell. Cyclic AMP binds to and stimulates protein kinase A (also called cyclic AMP–dependent protein kinase), which in turn attaches a phosphate group to (phosphorylates) specific amino acid groups of the calcium channel protein. Phosphorylation of the calcium channel is thought to be required for the channel to be able to open in response to depolarization, so an increase in cyclic AMP inside the cell translates into a greater number of openable calcium channels in the cell. In addition, each channel

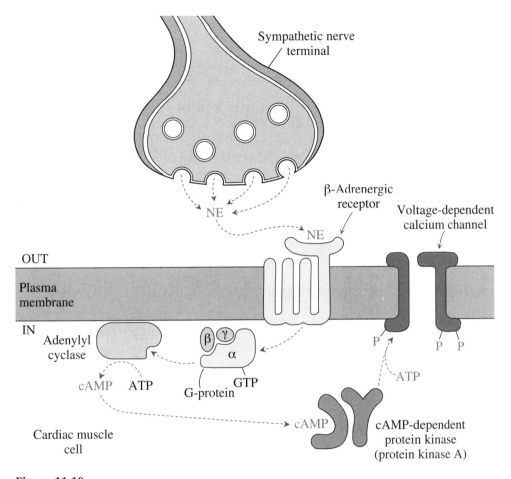

Figure 11-10
Norepinephrine promotes the activation of voltage-dependent calcium channels in cardiac muscle cells. When norepinephrine is released from the synaptic terminals of sympathetic neurons, it combines with β-adrenergic receptors in the postsynaptic membrane of the cardiac muscle cells. The activated receptor stimulates G-proteins that in turn activate adenylyl cyclase. This enzyme makes cyclic AMP from ATP. The cyclic AMP binds to and turns on protein kinase A, an enzyme that uses ATP as a phosphate donor to add a phosphate group to certain amino acids that are part of the calcium channel molecule. The phosphorylated calcium channel can be more readily opened upon depolarization and also remains open for a longer time. This increases the calcium influx during depolarization of the heart cell.

remains open for a longer time, on average, when it opens. Thus, phosphorylation of the channels greatly potentiates the inward calcium current that flows when the cardiac muscle cells are depolarized.

In the SA node, the triggering of the action potential depends on calcium channels. If there are more calcium channels available, the threshold potential for triggering the action potential will be lower and so the action potential will be triggered earlier during the pacemaker potential in the presence of norepinephrine. Outside of the SA node, in the muscle cells of the atria and ventricles, the role of the calcium channels is to produce the plateau phase of the action potential and to allow calcium influx, which contributes to the muscle contraction. An increase in the number of available calcium channels in these cells will increase the calcium influx during the plateau and thus increase the strength of contraction of the overall heart muscle. The combination of the increase in heart rate and the increase in strength of contraction makes the β-adrenergic receptors a powerful regulator of the amount of blood volume circulated per minute through the heart. The β-adrenergic receptors, which ultimately exert their effect by increasing the phosphorylation of voltage-activated calcium channels, are therefore targeted by many drugs that are used clinically to increase the heart output in human patients whose heart muscle has been damaged by disease.

One advantage of having the autonomic neurotransmitters exert their actions through G-protein–linked receptors, rather than by direct binding to ion channels, is that the nervous system can produce rather long-term effects on the ion channels of the heart without having to continuously provide an ongoing neural signal. Once the G-proteins are activated, they can affect channel activity for several seconds, until their activation terminates when GTP is hydrolyzed by the G-protein. Thus, acetylcholine can be released briefly from parasympathetic nerve terminals (or norepinephrine from sympathetic nerve terminals) and still affect the heart rate for several seconds after the acetylcholine stops being released. If, instead, acetylcholine bound to and opened a ligand-gated potassium channel in order to increase potassium permeability, the neurotransmitter would have to be continuously present, requiring the nervous system to continuously send signals from the central nervous system to the autonomic ganglia to produce a steady train of action potentials in the autonomic motor neurons. In the somatic nervous system, this is exactly what happens. Somatic motor neurons are tightly temporally coupled to the activation of their targets, the skeletal muscle fibers. This allows rapid, subsecond turning on and turning off of muscle activity under the control of the somatic nervous system. In general, the targets controlled by the autonomic nervous system are involved in much slower activities that are typically sustained for longer periods. Therefore, the slower and more sustained activation produced by indirect linkage between neurotransmitter receptor and ion channels seems well suited for the autonomic nervous system.

Summary

Motor systems of the nervous system can be divided into two parts, based on the motor targets that are innervated. The somatic nervous system is responsible for the control of the skeletal musculature, and thus for most of what we normally think of as the behavior of the organism. The autonomic nervous system is responsible for controlling other important organ systems involved in maintaining the internal homeostasis of the organism. The autonomic nervous system controls the cardiovascular system, the respiratory system, the digestive system, and so on. The autonomic nervous system is organized differently from the somatic nervous system. The motor neurons of the autonomic nervous system are located outside the central nervous system, in autonomic ganglia. The somatic motor neurons, by contrast, are located within the spinal cord and are thus part of the central nervous system. The autonomic nervous system is divided into the parasympathetic and the sympathetic divisions. The parasympathetic autonomic ganglia are located close to or in the target organs themselves. The sympathetic ganglia are typically located close to the central nervous system, and most of them are found in two chains of ganglia, called the paravertebral ganglia, that parallel the spinal column on each side of the spinal cord.

The nerve terminals of the parasympathetic postganglionic neurons release the neurotransmitter acetylcholine in the target organ. Acetylcholine typically acts on the target cells by activating muscarinic cholinergic receptors, which exert their postsynaptic actions by altering the level of internal second messengers, such as cyclic AMP, in the postsynaptic cell. The nerve terminals of the sympathetic postganglionic neurons release the transmitter norepinephrine, which also exerts its postsynaptic effect by altering the levels of internal second messengers. In organs that receive both sympathetic and parasympathetic innervation, the actions of acetylcholine and norepinephrine on the target cells are usually opposite. In the heart, for example, acetylcholine decreases heart rate and reduces cardiac output, while norepinephrine increases heart rate and cardiac output.

The muscle fibers making up the heart are specialized in a number of ways to carry out their function of efficiently pumping

Table 11-1 Comparison of some properties of skeletal and cardiac muscle fibers.

Property	Skeletal Muscle	Cardiac Muscle
Striated	Yes	Yes
Electrically coupled	No	Yes
Spontaneously contract in absence of nerve input	No	Yes
Duration of contraction controlled by duration of action potential	No	Yes
Action potential is similar to that of neurons	Yes	No
Calcium ions make an important contribution to the action potential	No	Yes
Effect of neural input	Excite	Excite or inhibit
Division of nervous system that provides neural control	Somatic	Autonomic (parasympathetic and sympathetic)
Neurotransmitter released onto muscle fibers by neurons	Acetylcholine	Acetylcholine (parasympathetic) or norepinephrine (sympathetic)
Effect of neurotransmitter on postsynaptic ion channels	Direct	Indirect (via G-proteins)

blood through the vessels of the circulatory system. These specializations lead to a number of differences between cardiac muscle fibers and skeletal muscle fibers, which are summarized in Table 11-1. In addition, the heart as an organ contains specific structures whose function is to coordinate the pumping activity. These structures include the SA node, the AV node, and the Purkinje fibers. The SA node is the master pacemaker region of the heart that controls the heart rate during normal physiological functioning of the heart. The AV node provides a path for electrical conduction between the atria and the ventricles and is responsible for the delay between atrial and ventricular contractions. The Purkinje fibers provide a rapidly conducting pathway for distributing excitation throughout the ventricles during the power stroke of a single heartbeat.

The activity of the heart is controlled by both the sympathetic and parasympathetic divisions of the autonomic nervous system. Acetylcholine released by the parasympathetic nerve terminals in the heart causes slowing of the heart rate by opening potassium channels. Norepinephrine released by the sympathetic nerve terminals increases the response of voltage-dependent calcium channels to depolarization, which increases the rate of beating and the strength of contraction. Both effects of neurotransmitters are indirect, mediated via receptors that act via GTP binding proteins.

These receptors are muscarinic receptors in the case of acetylcholine and β-adrenergic receptors in the case of norepinephrine. The effect of the β-adrenergic receptors is to increase the levels of cyclic AMP inside the cardiac cells, which in turn promotes phosphorylation of calcium channels by protein kinase A.

Derivation of the Nernst Equation

The Nernst equation is used extensively in the discussion of resting membrane potential and action potentials in this book. The derivation presented here is necessarily mathematical and requires some knowledge of differential and integral calculus to understand thoroughly. However, I have tried to explain the meaning of each step in words; hopefully, this will allow those without the necessary background to follow the logic qualitatively.

This derivation of the Nernst equation uses equations for the movement of ions down concentrational and electrical gradients to arrive at a quantitative description of the equilibrium condition. The starting point is the realization that at equilibrium there will be no net movement of the ion across the membrane. In the presence of both concentration and electrical gradients, this means that the rate of movement of the ion down the concentration gradient is equal and opposite to the rate of movement of the ion down the electrical gradient. For a charged substance (an ion), movement across the membrane constitutes a transmembrane electrical current, I. Thus, at equilibrium

$$I_C = -I_E \qquad \text{(A-1)}$$

or

$$I_C + I_E = 0 \qquad \text{(A-2)}$$

where I_C and I_E are the currents due to the concentrational and electrical gradients, respectively.

Concentrational Flux

Consider first the current due to the concentration gradient, which is given by

$$I_C = A\Phi_C ZF \qquad (A\text{-}3)$$

In words, Equation (A-3) states that the current through the membrane of area A will be equal to the flux, Φ_C, of the ion down the concentration gradient (number of ions per second per unit area of membrane) multiplied by Z (the valence of the ion) and F (Faraday's constant; 96,500 coulombs per mole of univalent ion). The factor ZF translates the flux of ions into flux of charge and hence into an electrical current. The flux Φ_C for a given ion (call the ion Y, for example) will depend on the concentration gradient of Y across the membrane (that is, $[Y]_{in} - [Y]_{out}$) and on the membrane permeability to Y, p_Y. Quantitatively, this relation is given by

$$\Phi_C = p_Y \, ([Y]_{in} - [Y]_{out}) \qquad (A\text{-}4)$$

Note that p_Y has units of velocity (cm/sec), in order for Φ_C to have units of molecules/sec/cm^2 (remember that $[Y]$ has units of molecules/cm^3). The permeability coefficient, p_Y, is in turn given by

$$p_Y = D_Y \, /a \qquad (A\text{-}5)$$

where D_Y is the diffusion constant for Y within the membrane and a is the thickness of the membrane. D_Y can be expanded to yield

$$D_Y = uRT \qquad (A\text{-}6)$$

where u is the mobility of the ion within the membrane and RT (the gas constant times the absolute temperature) is the thermal energy available to drive ion movement. Substituting Equation (A-6) in (A-5) and the result in Equation (A-4) yields

$$\Phi_C a = uRT([Y]_{in} - [Y]_{out}) \qquad (A\text{-}7)$$

Equation (A-7) gives us the flux through a membrane of thickness a, but we would like a more general expression that gives us the flux through any arbitrary plane in the presence of a concentration gradient. To arrive at this expression, consider the situation

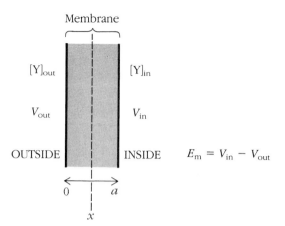

diagrammed in Figure A-1, which shows a segment of membrane separating two compartments. The dimension perpendicular to the membrane is called x, and the membrane extends from zero to a (thickness = a). In this situation, Equation (A-7) can be expressed in the form of an integral equation:

$$\Phi_C\left(\int_0^a dx\right) = uRT\left(\int_0^a dC\right) \qquad \text{(A-8)}$$

Here, C stands for the concentration of the ion; therefore, in reference to Figure A-1, C_a is $[Y]_{in}$ and C_0 is $[Y]_{out}$. Differentiating both sides of Equation (A-8) yields

$$\Phi_c \, dx = uRT \, dC \qquad \text{(A-9)}$$

which can be arranged to give the more general form of Equation (A-7) that we desire:

$$\Phi_C = uRT \, (dC/dx) \qquad \text{(A-10)}$$

Equation (A-10) can be substituted into Equation (A-3) to give us the ionic current due to the concentration gradient.

Current Due to Electrical Gradient

Return now to the current driven by the electrical gradient, which can be expressed

$$I_E = A\Phi_E ZF \tag{A-11}$$

The flux, Φ_E, of a charged particle through a plane at position x in the presence of a voltage gradient dV/dx will be

$$\Phi_E = uZFC\,(dV/dx) \tag{A 12}$$

Again, u is the mobility of the ion, and C is the concentration of the ion at position x. The factor ZFC is then the concentration of charge at the location of the plane; this is necessary because the voltage gradient dV/dx acts on charge and ZFC gives the "concentration" of charge at position $= x$. Equation (A-12) is analogous to Equation (A-10), except it is the voltage gradient rather than the concentration gradient that is of interest.

Total Current at Equilibrium

Equations (A-12), (A-11), (A-10), and (A-3) can be combined into the form of Equation (A-2) to give

$$uAZF\left(RT\frac{dc}{dx} + ZFC\frac{dV}{dx} \right) = 0 \tag{A-13}$$

This requires that

$$RT\left(\frac{dC}{dx}\right) = -ZFC\left(\frac{dV}{dx}\right) \tag{A-14}$$

Equation (A-14) can be rearranged to give a differential equation that can be solved for the equilibrium voltage gradient:

$$\left(-\frac{RT}{ZF}\right)\left(\frac{dC}{C}\right) = dV \tag{A-15}$$

This can be solved for V by integrating across the membrane. Using the nomenclature of Figure A-1, the integrals are

$$-\frac{RT}{ZF}\int_{[Y]_{out}}^{[Y]_{in}} \frac{dC}{C} = \int_{V_{out}}^{V_{in}} dV \tag{A-16}$$

The solution to these definite integrals is

$$-\frac{RT}{ZF}(\ln[Y]_{in} - \ln[Y]_{out}) = V_{in} - V_{out} \qquad \text{(A-17)}$$

or

$$\frac{RT}{ZF}\ln\left(\frac{[Y]_{out}}{[Y]_{in}}\right) = V_{in} - V_{out} = E_M \qquad \text{(A-18)}$$

Equation (A-18) is the Nernst equation.

Derivation of the Goldman Equation

The Goldman equation, or constant-field equation, is important to an understanding of the factors that govern the steady-state membrane potential. As discussed in Chapter 4, the Goldman equation describes the nonequilibrium membrane potential reached when two or more ions with unequal equilibrium potentials are free to move across the membrane. The basic strategy in this derivation is to use the flux equations derived in Appendix A to solve separately for the ionic current carried by each permeant ion and then to set the sum of all ionic currents equal to zero. The derivation is somewhat more complex than that of the Nernst equation in Appendix A, and it requires some knowledge of differential and integral calculus to follow in detail. Nevertheless, it should be possible for those without the necessary mathematics to follow the logic of the steps and thus to gain some insight into the physical mechanisms described by the equation.

When several ions are moving across the membrane simultaneously, a steady value of membrane potential will be reached when the sum of the ionic currents carried by the individual ions is zero; that is, for permeant ions A, B, and C

$$I_A + I_B + I_C = 0 \tag{B-1}$$

The first step in arriving at a value of membrane potential that satisfies this condition is to solve for the net ionic flux, Φ, for each ion separately. The total flux for a particular ion will be the sum of the flux due to the concentration gradient and the flux due to the electrical gradient:

$$\Phi_T = \Phi_C + \Phi_V \tag{B-2}$$

The expressions for Φ_C and Φ_V are given by Equations (A-10) and (A-12) in Appendix A. Thus, Equation (B-2) becomes

$$\Phi_T = uRT\ (dC/dx) + uZFC\ (dV/dx) \tag{B-3}$$

If it is assumed that the electric field across the membrane is constant (this is the constant-field assumption from which the equation draws its alternative name) and that the thickness of the membrane is a, then

$$dV/dx = V/a \tag{B-4}$$

In that case, Equation (B-3) can be written

$$\frac{\Phi_T}{uRT} = \frac{dC}{dx} + \frac{ZFV}{RTa}C \tag{B-5}$$

This is a differential equation of the form

$$Q = \frac{dC}{dx} + P(x)C$$

which has a solution

$$C \exp\left(\int P(x)dx\right) = \int Q \exp\left(\int P(x)dx\right)dx + \text{constant} \tag{B-6}$$

In this instance, $Q = \Phi_T/(uRT)$ and $P(x) = (ZFV)/(RTa)$. Making these substitutions and integrating Equation (B-6) across the membrane of thickness a (that is, from zero to a) gives

$$C \exp\left(\frac{ZFV}{RTa}\right)\Bigg|_0^a = \frac{\Phi_T}{uRT}\int_0^a \exp\left(\frac{ZFVx}{RTa}\right)dx \tag{B-7}$$

This becomes

$$C_a \exp\left(\frac{ZFV}{RT}\right) - C_0 = \frac{\Phi_T}{uRT}\left[\exp\left(\frac{ZFVx}{RTa}\right)\Big/\left(\frac{ZFV}{RTa}\right)\right]\Bigg|_0^a$$

or

$$C_a \exp\left(\frac{ZFV}{RT}\right) - C_0 = \frac{\Phi_T}{uRT}\frac{RTa}{ZFV}\left[\exp\left(\frac{ZFVa}{RTa}\right) - \exp\left(\frac{ZFV \cdot 0}{RTa}\right)\right]$$

Rearranging and combining terms yields

$$C_a \exp\left(\frac{ZFV}{RT}\right) - C_0 = \frac{\Phi_T a}{uZFV}\left[\exp\left(\frac{ZFV}{RT}\right) - 1\right]$$

This can be solved for Φ_T to yield

$$\Phi_T = \frac{uZFV}{a}\left[\frac{C_a \exp(ZFV/RT) - C_0}{\exp(ZFV/RT) - 1}\right] \tag{B-8}$$

Now, C_a and C_0 are the concentrations of the ion just within the membrane. These concentrations are related to the concentrations in the fluids inside and outside the cell by $C_a = \beta C_{in}$ and $C_0 = \beta C_{out}$, where β is the oil–water partition coefficient for the ion in question. Substituting these in Equation (B-8) gives

$$\Phi_T = \frac{\beta uZFV}{a}\left[\frac{C_{in} \exp(ZFV/RT) - C_{out}}{\exp(ZFV/RT) - 1}\right] \tag{B-9}$$

The permeability constant, p_i, for a particular ion is given by $p_i = \beta uRT/a$, or $p_i/RT = \beta u/a$. Making this substitution in Equation (B-9) gives

$$\Phi_T = \frac{p_i ZFV}{RT}\left[\frac{C_{in} \exp(ZFV/RT) - C_{out}}{\exp(ZFV/RT) - 1}\right] \tag{B-10}$$

The flux, Φ_T, for an ion can be converted to a flow of electrical current, as required in Equation (B-1), by multiplying by ZF (the number of coulombs per mole of ion); therefore

$$I = \frac{p_i Z^2 F^2 V}{RT}\left[\frac{C_{in} \exp(ZFV/RT) - C_{out}}{\exp(ZFV/RT) - 1}\right] \tag{B-11}$$

This is the expression we need for each ion in Equation (B-1). For instance, if the three permeant ions are Na, K, and Cl with permeabilities p_{Na}, p_K, and p_{Cl}, then Equation (B-1) becomes (keeping in mind that the valence of chloride is -1)

$$\frac{F^2 V}{RT} \left[\frac{p_{\rm K}([{\rm K}]_{\rm in} e^{FV/RT} - [{\rm K}]_{\rm out}) + p_{\rm Na}([{\rm Na}]_{\rm in} e^{FV/RT} - [{\rm Na}]_{\rm out})}{\exp(FV/RT) - 1} + \frac{p_{\rm Cl}([{\rm Cl}]_{\rm in} e^{-FV/RT} - [{\rm Cl}]_{\rm out})}{\exp(-FV/RT) - 1} \right] = 0$$

Multiplying through by $-\exp(FV/RT)/-\exp(FV/RT)$ and rearranging yields

$$\frac{F^2 V}{RT(\exp(FV/RT) - 1)} [(p_{\rm K}[{\rm K}]_{\rm in} + p_{\rm Na}[{\rm Na}]_{\rm in} + p_{\rm Cl}[{\rm Cl}]_{\rm out}) e^{FV/RT} - (p_{\rm K}[{\rm K}]_{\rm out} + p_{\rm Na}[{\rm Na}]_{\rm out} + p_{\rm Cl}[{\rm Cl}]_{\rm in})] = 0$$

This requires that

$$(p_{\rm K}[{\rm K}]_{\rm in} + p_{\rm Na}[{\rm Na}]_{\rm in} + p_{\rm Cl}[{\rm Cl}]_{\rm out}) e^{FV/RT} - (p_{\rm K}[{\rm K}]_{\rm out} + p_{\rm Na}[{\rm Na}]_{\rm out} + p_{\rm Cl}[{\rm Cl}]_{\rm in}) = 0$$

or

$$e^{FV/RT} = \frac{(p_{\rm K}[{\rm K}]_{\rm out} + p_{\rm Na}[{\rm Na}]_{\rm out} + p_{\rm Cl}[{\rm Cl}]_{\rm in})}{(p_{\rm K}[{\rm K}]_{\rm in} + p_{\rm Na}[{\rm Na}]_{\rm in} + p_{\rm Cl}[{\rm Cl}]_{\rm out})}$$

Taking the natural logarithm of both sides and solving for V yields the usual form of the Goldman equation

$$V = \frac{RT}{F} \ln\left(\frac{p_{\rm K}[{\rm K}]_{\rm out} + p_{\rm Na}[{\rm Na}]_{\rm out} + p_{\rm Cl}[{\rm Cl}]_{\rm in}}{p_{\rm K}[{\rm K}]_{\rm in} + p_{\rm Na}[{\rm Na}]_{\rm in} + p_{\rm Cl}[{\rm Cl}]_{\rm out}} \right)$$

Suggested Readings

This section contains suggested additional readings for those interested in obtaining more advanced information about the topics covered in this book or in reading additional introductory material. The references are divided into two sections: General References, which present more advanced information, and Specific Topics. The references given under Specific Topics represent a range of difficulty from introductory to original papers in technical journals.

Rating system
(*) Introductory level; for a general, nonscientist audience or beginning students
(**) Intermediate level; a general review for nonspecialists or second-level students
(***) Advanced level; for advanced students wishing greater detail
(****) Original research articles; usually intended for specialists working in the field

General References

Aidley, D. J. *The Physiology of Excitable Cells.* 2nd ed. New York: Cambridge University Press, 1979. (**)

Annual Review of Physiology, Annual Review of Neuroscience, and Annual Review of Biophysics and Bioengineering. Published yearly by Annual Reviews, Inc., Palo Alto, Calif. Each volume contains review articles covering recent developments in physiology and neuroscience. Intended for working scientists in the field. Typically requires good background knowledge. (**) – (***)

Davson, H. *A Textbook of General Physiology.* 4th ed. Boston: Little, Brown, 1970. (***)

Guyton, A. C. *Textbook of Medical Physiology*. 6th ed. Philadelphia: Saunders, 1981. (**)

Hall, J. W. (ed.) *An Introduction to Molecular Neurobiology*. Sunderland, Mass.: Sinauer, 1992. (**)

Handbook of Physiology. Volumes published periodically by the American Physiological Society. Those on neurophysiology and cardiovascular physiology contain advanced material on topics covered in this book. Articles often require advanced knowledge of biology, chemistry, and mathematics. (***) – (****)

Hille, B. *Ionic Channels of Excitable Membranes*. 2nd ed. Sunderland, Mass.: Sinauer Associates, 1992. (***)

Jack, J. J. B., Noble, D., and Tsien, R. W. *Electric Current Flow in Excitable Cells*. New York: Oxford University Press, 1983. Not for the timid. Only those who are comfortable with partial differential equations, complex numbers, and Laplace transforms should trespass here. (****)

Kandel, E. R., Schwartz, J. H., and Jessell, T. M. (eds.) *Principles of Neural Science*. New York: Elsevier, 1991. (***)

Katz, B. *Nerve, Muscle and Synapse*. New York: McGraw-Hill, 1966. (**)

Levitan, I. B., and Kaczmarek, L. K. *The Neuron, Cell and Molecular Biology*. New York: Oxford University Press, 1991. (**)

Mountcastle, V. B. *Medical Physiology*. 14th ed. St. Louis: C. V. Mosby, 1979. (**)

Physiological Reviews. This journal is published quarterly by the American Physiological Society. Issues often contain reviews of recent advances in nerve and muscle physiology. (***) – (****)

Ruch, T. C., and Patton, H. D. *Physiology and Biophysics*. 20th ed. St. Louis: C.V. Mosby, 1974. (***)

Specific Topics

The Cell and Its Composition

Bretscher, M. S. The molecules of the cell membrane. *Scientific American* 253(1985):100. (*)

Burton, R. F. The composition of animal cells: solutes contributing to osmotic pressure and charge balance. *Comparative Biochemistry and Physiology [B]* 76(1983):663. (****)

Fettiplace, R., and Haydon, D. A. Water permeability of lipid membranes *Physiological Reviews* 60(1980):510. (***)

Folsome, C. E. *Life: Origin and Evolution*. San Francisco: Freeman, 1979. A collection of *Scientific American* reprints. (*)

Gilles, R. *Mechanisms of Osmoregulation: Maintenance of Cell Volume*. New York: Wiley, 1979. (***)

Kwon, H. M., and Handler, J. S. Cell volume regulated transporters of compatible osmolytes. *Current Opinion in Cell Biology* 7(1995):465. (**)

Macknight, A. D. Principles of cell volume regulation. *Renal Physiology and Biochemistry* 11(1988):114. (***)

MacKnight, A. D. C., and Leaf, A. Regulation of cellular volume. *Physiological Reviews* 57(1977):510. (***)

Orgel, L. E. The origin of life on the earth. *Scientific American* 271(1994): 76. (*)

Potts, W. T. Osmotic and ionic regulation. *Annual Review of Physiology* 30(1968):73. (***)

Singer, S. J. The molecular organization of membranes. *Annual Review of Biochemistry* 43(1974):805. (**)

Stein, W. D. *The Movement of Molecules Across Cell Membranes.* New York: Academic Press, 1967. (***)

Verkman, A. S. Water channels in cell membranes. *Annual Review of Physiology* 54(1992):97. (***)

Resting Membrane Potential

Glynn, I. M. How does the sodium pump pump? *Society of General Physiologists Series* 43(1988):1. (***)

Hille, B. *Ionic Channels of Excitable Membranes.* 2nd ed. Sunderland, Mass.: Sinauer Associates, 1992. (***)

Hodgkin, A. L., and Horowicz, P. The influence of potassium and chloride ions on the membrane potential of single muscle fibers. *Journal of Physiology* 148(1959)127. (****)

Hodgkin, A. L., and Katz, B. The effects of sodium ions on the electrical activity of the giant axon of the squid. *Journal of Physiology* 108 (1949):37. (****)

Hodgkin, A. L., and Keynes, R. D. Active transport of cations in giant axons from *Sepia* and *Loligo. Journal of Physiology* 128(1955):28. (****)

Kaplan, J. H. Ion movements through the sodium pump. *Annual Review of Physiology* 47(1985):535. (***)

Katz, B. *Nerve, Muscle and Synapse.* New York: McGraw-Hill, 1966. (*)

Keynes, R. D. Ion channels in the nerve cell membrane. *Scientific American* 240(1979):126. (*)

Neher, E., and Sakmann, B. (eds.) *Single Channel Recording.* 2nd ed. New York: Plenum Press, 1995. (****)

Sather, W. A., Yang, J., and Tsien, R. W. Structural basis of ion channel permeation and selectivity. *Current Opinion in Neurobiology* 4(1994): 313. (**)

Thomas, R. C. Electrogenic sodium pump in nerve and muscle cells. *Physiological Reviews* 52(1972):563. (***)

Wallick, E. T., Lane, L. K., and Schwartz, A. Biochemical mechanism of the sodium pump. *Annual Review of Physiology* 41(1979):397. (***)

Action Potential

Armstrong, C. M. Voltage-dependent ion channels and their gating. *Physiological Reviews* 72(1992):S5. (***)

Baker, P. F. The nerve axon. *Scientific American* 214(1966):74. (*)

Bezanilla, F., and Stefani, E. Voltage-dependent gating of ionic channels. *Annual Review of Biophysics and Biomolecular Structure* 23(1994):819. (****)

Catterall, W. A. Cellular and molecular biology of voltage-gated sodium channels. *Physiological Reviews* 72(1992):S15. (***)

Catterall, W. A. Structure and function of voltage-gated ion channels. *Annual Review of Biochemistry* 64(1995):493. (***)

Hille, B. *Ionic Channels of Excitable Membranes.* 2nd ed. Sunderland, Mass.: Sinauer Associates, 1992. (***)

Hodgkin, A. L. *The Conduction of the Nervous Impulse.* Springfield, Ill.: Thomas, 1963. (***)

Hodgkin, A. L., and Huxley, A. F. Currents carried by sodium and potassium ions through the membrane of the giant axon of *Loligo. Journal of Physiology* 116(1952):449. (****)

Hodgkin, A. L., and Huxley, A. F. The components of membrane conductance in the giant axon of *Loligo. Journal of Physiology* 116(1952): 473. (****)

Hodgkin, A. L., and Huxley, A. F. The dual effect of membrane potential on sodium conductance in the giant axon of *Loligo. Journal of Physiology* 116(1952):497. (****)

Hodgkin, A. L., and Huxley, A. F. Quantitative description of membrane current and its application to conduction and excitation in nerve. *Journal of Physiology* 117(1952):500. (****)

Hodgkin, A. L., and Huxley, A. F. Movement of sodium and potassium ions during nervous activity. *Cold Spring Harbor Symposia on Quantitative Biology* 17(1952):43. A brief, simplified account of the results of the voltage-clamp experiments on the squid giant axon. (*)

Kallen, R. G., Cohen, S. A.,and Barchi, R. L. Structure, function, and expression of voltage-dependent sodium channels. *Molecular Neurobiology* 7(1993):383. (**)

Morell, P., and Norton, W. T. Myelin. *Scientific American* 242(1980):88, 92, 96. (*)

Neher, E., and Sakmann, B. The patch clamp technique. *Scientific American* 266(1992):28. (*)

Pallotta, B. S., and Wagoner, P. K. Voltage-dependent potassium channels since Hodgkin and Huxley. *Physiological Reviews* 72(1992):S49. (***)

Stevens, C. F. The neuron. *Scientific American* 241(1979):54. (*)

Tasaki, I. Conduction of impulses in the myelinated nerve fiber. *Cold Spring Harbor Symposia on Quantitative Biology* 17(1952):37. (****)

Waxman, S. G., and Ritchie, J. M. Molecular dissection of the myelinated axon. *Annals of Neurology* 33(1993):121. (***)

Synaptic Transmission

Augustine, G. J., Burns, M. E., DeBello, W. M., Pettit, D. L., and Schweizer, F. E. Exocytosis—proteins and perturbations. *Annual Review of Pharmacology and Toxicology* 36(1996):659. (***)

Augustine, G. J., Charlton, M. P., and Smith, S. J. Calcium action in synaptic transmitter release. *Annual Review of Neuroscience* 10(1987):633. (***)

Axelrod, J. Neurotransmitters. *Scientific American* 230(1974):59. (*)

Bennett, M. K., and Scheller, R. H. A molecular description of synaptic vesicle membrane trafficking. *Annual Review of Biochemistry* 63(1994): 63. (***)

Bertolino, M., and Llinas, R. R. The central role of voltage-activated and receptor-activated calcium channels in neuronal cells. *Annual Review of Pharmacology and Toxicology* 32(1992):399. (***)

Brown, D. A. G-proteins and potassium currents in neurons. *Annual Review of Physiology* 52(1990):215. (***)

Calakos, N., and Scheller, R. H. Synaptic vesicle biogenesis, docking, and fusion—a molecular description. *Physiological Reviews* 76(1996):1. (***)

Catterall, W. A. Molecular properties of a superfamily of plasma-membrane cation channels. *Current Opinion in Cell Biology* 6(1994):607. (**)

Ceccarelli, B., and Hurlbut, W. P. Vesicle hypothesis of the release of acetylcholine. *Physiological Reviews* 60(1980):396. (**)

Clapham, D. E. Direct G protein activation of ion channels? *Annual Review of Neuroscience* 17(1994):441. (***)

Coombs, J. S., Eccles, J. C., and Fatt, P. Excitatory synaptic action in motoneurones. *Journal of Physiology* 130(1955):374. (****)

Del Castillo, J., and Katz, B. Quantal components of the end-plate potential. *Journal of Physiology* 124(1954):560. (****)

De Robertis, E. Ultrastructure and cytochemistry of the synaptic region. *Science* 156(1967):907. (*)

Fatt, P., and Katz, B. Spontaneous subthreshold activity at motor nerve endings. *Journal of Physiology* 117(1952):109. (****)

Gilman, A. G. G proteins: transducers of receptor-generated signals. *Annual Review of Biochemistry* 56(1987):615. (**)

Hamm, H. E., and Gilchrist, A. Heterotrimeric G proteins. *Current Opinion in Cell Biology* 8(1996):189. (**)

Heuser, J. E. Review of electron microscopic evidence favoring vesicle exocytosis as the structural basis for quantal release during synaptic transmission. *Quarterly Journal of Experimental Physiology* 74(1989):1051. (***)

Heuser, J. E., and Reese, T. S. Structural changes after transmitter release at the frog neuromuscular junction. *Journal of Cell Biology* 88(1981):564. (****)

Jahn, R., and Sudhof, T. C. Synaptic vesicles and exocytosis. *Annual Review of Neuroscience* 17(1994):219. (**)

Katz, B. Quantal mechanism of neural transmitter release. *Science* 173(1971):123. (*)

Katz, B., and Miledi, R. The timing of calcium action during neuromuscular transmission. *Journal of Physiology* 189(1967):535. (****)

Kennedy, M. B. The biochemistry of synaptic regulation in the central nervous system. *Annual Review of Biochemistry* 63(1994):571. (***)

Lester, H. A. The response to acetylcholine. *Scientific American* 236 (1977):106, 118. (*)

Levitan, I. B. Modulation of ion channels by protein phosphorylation and dephosphorylation. *Annual Review of Physiology* 56(1994):193. (**)

Linder, M. E., and Gilman, A. G. G proteins. *Scientific American* 267 (1992):56. (*)

MacDonald, R. L., and Olsen, R. W. GABA$_A$ receptor channels. *Annual Review of Neuroscience* 17(1994):569. (***)

Matthews, G. Neurotransmitter release. *Annual Review of Neuroscience* 19(1996):219. (***)

Matthews, G., and Wickelgren, W. O. Glycine, GABA and synaptic inhibition of reticulospinal neurones of lamprey. *Journal of Physiology* 293(1979):393. (****)

Matthews, G., and Wickelgren, W. O. Glutamate and synaptic excitation of reticulospinal neurones of lamprey. *Journal of Physiology* 293(1979): 417. (****)

Nicholls, D. G. *Proteins, Transmitters and Synapses.* Oxford: Blackwell Scientific, 1994. (**)

Tsien, R. W., Lipscombe, D., Madison, D., Bley, K., and Fox, A. Reflections on Ca^{2+}-channel diversity, 1988-1994. *Trends in Neurosciences* 18 (1995):52. (**)

Van der Kloot, W., and Molgo, J. Quantal acetylcholine release at the vertebrate neuromuscular junction. *Physiological Reviews* 74(1994):899. (***)

Wickman, K., and Clapham, D. E. Ion channel regulation by G proteins. *Physiological Reviews* 75(1995):865. (***)

Skeletal Muscle

Ashley, C. C., and Ridgeway, E. B. Simultaneous recording of membrane potential, calcium transient and tension in single muscle fibres. *Nature* 219(1968):1168. (****)

Bourne, G. H. *The Structure and Function of Muscle.* 2nd ed. New York: Academic Press, 1972 (Vol. I), 1973 (Vols. II and III), 1974 (Vol. IV). (***)

Buchtal, F., and Schmalbruch, H. Motor unit of mammalian muscle. *Physiological Reviews* 60(1980):90. (***)

Caputo, C. Excitation and contraction processes in muscle. *Annual Review of Biophysics and Bioengineering* 7(1978):63. (***)

Cohen, C. The protein switch of muscle contraction. *Scientific American* 233(1975):36. (*)

Endo, M. Calcium release from the sarcoplasmic reticulum. *Physiological Reviews* 57(1977):71. (***)

Freund, H.-J. Motor unit and muscle activity in voluntary motor control. *Physiological Reviews* 63(1983):387. (***)

Hoyle, G. How is muscle turned on and off? *Scientific American* 222 (1970):84. (*)

Hoyle, G. *Muscles and Their Neural Control.* New York: Wiley, 1983. (**)

Huxley, H. E. The structural basis of muscular contraction. *Proceedings of the Royal Society of London Series B* 178(1971):131. (***)

Huxley, H. E. Muscular contraction and cell motility. *Nature* 243(1973): 445. (**)

Huxley, H. E. A personal view of muscle and motility mechanisms. *Annual Review of Physiology* 58(1996):1. (**)

Schneider, M. F. Control of calcium release in functioning skeletal muscle fibers. *Annual Review of Physiology* 56(1994):463. (***)

Sheterline, P. *Mechanism of Cell Motility: Molecular Aspects of Contractility.* New York: Academic Press, 1983. (***)

Stracher, A. *Muscle and Nonmuscle Motility.* Vol. I. New York: Academic Press, 1983. (**)

Heart

Adolph, E. F. The heart's pacemaker. *Scientific American* 216(1967):32. (*)

Brown, H. F. Electrophysiology of the sinoatrial node. *Physiological Reviews* 62(1982):505. (***)

Campbell, D. L., Rasmusson, R. L., and Strauss, H. C. Ionic current mechanisms generating vertebrate primary cardiac pacemaker activity at the single cell level: an integrative view. *Annual Review of Physiology* 54(1992):279. (***)

Carpenter, D. O. *Cellular Pacemakers.* Vol. 1. New York: Wiley, 1982. (**)

Clapham, D. E. Direct G protein activation of ion channels? *Annual Review of Neuroscience* 17(1994):441. (***)

Deal, K. K., England, S. K., and Tamkun, M. M. Molecular physiology of cardiac potassium channels. *Physiological Reviews* 76(1996):49. (***)

Fozzard, H. A. Heart: excitation-contraction coupling. *Annual Review of Physiology* 39(1977):201. (***)

Gilman, A. G. G proteins: transducers of receptor-generated signals. *Annual Review of Biochemistry* 56(1987):615. (***)

Hartzell, H. C. Regulation of cardiac ion channels by catecholamines, acetylcholine and second messenger systems. *Progress in Biophysics and Molecular Biology* 52(1988):165. (***)

Hartzell, H. C., Méry, P.-F., Fischmeister, R., and Szabo, G. Sympathetic regulation of cardiac calcium current is due exclusively to cAMP-dependent phosphorylation. *Nature* 351(1991):573. (****)

Irisawa, H., Brown, H. F., and Giles, W. Cardiac pacemaking in the sinoatrial node. *Physiological Reviews* 73(1993):197.(***)

Kobilka, B. Adrenergic receptors as models for G protein-coupled receptors. *Annual Review of Neuroscience* 15(1992):87. (***)

Linder, M. E., and Gilman, A. G. G proteins. *Scientific American* 267 (1992):56. (*)

Noble, D. *The Initiation of the Heartbeat.* 2nd ed. New York: Oxford University Press, 1979. (***)

Szabo, G., and Otero, A. S. G protein mediated regulation of K^+ channels in heart. *Annual Review of Physiology* 52(1990):293. (***)

Wickman, K., and Clapham, D. E. Ion channel regulation by G proteins. *Physiological Reviews* 75(1995):865. (***)

Note: Page numbers followed by f refer to illustrations; page numbers followed by t refer to tables.